SMARTCLIP™
SELF-LIGATING APPLIANCE SYSTEM

Commissioning Editor: *Michael Parkinson*

Development Editor: *Barbara Simmons*

Copy Editor: *Lotika Singha*

Project Manager: *Andrew Palfreyman*

Designer: *Stewart Larking*

SMARTCLIP™
SELF-LIGATING APPLIANCE SYSTEM
CONCEPT AND BIOMECHANICS

HUGO TREVISI

Orthodontist, Presidente Prudente, Brazil

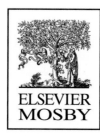

EDINBURGH LONDON NEW YORK OXFORD PHILADELPHIA ST LOUIS SYDNEY TORONTO 2007

ELSEVIER
MOSBY

MOSBY

An imprint of Elsevier Limited

First published 2007
Reprinted 2008

ISBN: 978-0-7234-3395-8

British Library Cataloguing in Publication Data
A catalogue record for this book is available from the British Library

Library of Congress Cataloging in Publication Data
A catalog record for this book is available from the Library of Congress

Notice
Knowledge and best practice in this field are constantly changing. As new research and experience broaden our knowledge, changes in practice, treatment and drug therapy may become necessary or appropriate. Readers are advised to check the most current information provided (i) on procedures featured or (ii) by the manufacturer of each product to be administered, to verify the recommended dose or formula, the method and duration of administration, and contraindications. It is the responsibility of the practitioner, relying on their own experience and knowledge of the patient, to make diagnoses, to determine dosages and the best treatment for each individual patient, and to take all appropriate safety precautions. To the fullest extent of the law, neither the Publisher nor the Author assumes any liability for any injury and/or damage to persons or property arising out or related to any use of the material contained in this book.

The Publisher

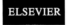 your source for books, journals and multimedia in the health sciences
www.elsevierhealth.com

Working together to grow libraries in developing countries
www.elsevier.com | www.bookaid.org | www.sabre.org
ELSEVIER   BOOK AID International   Sabre Foundation

The publisher's policy is to use **paper manufactured from sustainable forests**

08 09 10 10 9 8 7 6 5 4 3 2

Typeset by IMH(Cartrif), Loanhead, Scotland
Printed in Spain

Foreword

It was four years ago when the notion of integrating MBT™ System principles and mechanics with self-ligating appliances was presented to the three of us (McLaughlin, Bennett and Trevisi). Two years earlier we had collectively published the defining text on the MBT™ philosophy of treatment, *Systemized Orthodontic Treatment Mechanics*. We had spent many years developing the appliance and the methods on a solid base of clinical evidence. Although we were (and are) committed to continuous improvement and an evolution of the appliance, we were cautious about folding this relatively new approach into our core philosophy. During this meeting in 2003, Dr Trevisi agreed to be our MBT™ system representative and was charged with the responsibility of understanding the intricacies and potential benefits of this new low-friction approach when coupled with the tenants of MBT™ system mechanics. During the past four years, Hugo worked in his clinic in Presidente Prudente, Brazil, and with the product development team in Monrovia, California, toward that goal. This impressive text is a comprehensive presentation of his work and his successful integration of the MBT™ System approach with self-ligating mechanics. The results are excellent.

Richard P McLaughlin

Preface

At the beginning of the twentieth century, Edward Angle presented a new fixed orthodontic appliance: the Edgewise Appliance. This innovative device allowed tooth control in three dimensions: it controlled the angulation, inclination and rotation of teeth. Such an achievement was made possible due to the new features of this unique device – square brackets, a horizontal slot and brackets soldered to the buccal face of the metal bands. During its evolution this appliance received twin wings to allow better tying-in of the wires to the bracket slot, which led to improved three-dimensional control during tooth movement.

During the 1930s, 1940s, and 1950s, the Edgewise Appliance system was overwhelmingly successful as a result of the three-dimensional control of the teeth, although the ideal positioning of teeth was only obtained by inserting first, second and third order bends in the orthodontic archwires. In the 1960s, new studies were conducted on tooth positioning using fixed appliances. The aim was to allow the brackets to control the three-dimensional movements of the teeth.

In the 1970s, Lawrence F Andrews introduced a new generation of orthodontic appliances with his Straight-Wire™ Appliance. The development of this appliance was built on an analysis of 120 non-orthodontic normal cases. The Straight-Wire™ Appliance had the same features as the Edgewise Appliance, such as square- and rectangular-shaped brackets and an .022/.028 slot size. However, some new features were introduced, such as angulation built into the mesial and distal wings, torque in the base, rotation for canines and second premolars in the base of the mesial

and distal slot, and molar rotation obtained by adding metal to the distal end of the buccal tubes.

Again, in the 1990s, a new advancement in orthodontics took place with the development of rhomboidal-shaped twin bracket preadjusted appliances. In these brackets, the angulation imparted to the teeth was included in the bracket design.

By the end of the 1990s, based on their 20 years of experience working with preadjusted appliances, McLaughlin, Bennett and Trevisi introduced a range of improvements and specification changes to improve the three-dimensional control of teeth when working with preadjusted appliances. The authors proposed increasing the torque for upper incisors, decreasing the torque for the lower incisors, the use of three torque options for the canines, increasing the negative torque for the upper molars and reducing the negative torque from lower canines to second molars. All these improvements were based on sliding mechanics, applying light force levels, use of the .022/.028 slot size and .019/.025 archwires. All aspects of this treatment approach were published in 2001 in the textbook entitled *Systemized Orthodontic Treatment Mechanics*. These new improvements and specification changes were welcomed by clinicians worldwide.

By this time although fixed appliance had been used for orthodontic treatment for almost a century, and many improvements had been made, orthodontic appliances continued to be ligated appliances. Despite the medium-sized, twin edgewise bracket system having proved its reliability, it still has a disadvantage, the friction caused by metal or elastic ligatures holding the archwire in the bracket slot during the three stages of the orthodontic treatment – aligning, leveling and space closure.

Considering all the issues mentioned above, a new design has been introduced for preadjusted appliances – an orthodontic appliance that continues to be a twin appliance system with rhomboidal shape and .022/.028 slot but is capable of decreasing the friction between the bracket slot and the archwire, and thus reducing the levels of applied force. This new appliance, called the SmartClip™ Self-Ligating Appliance System, also has features as the previous existing appliances, providing easy handling for the professional and comfort for the patient.

While incorporating all the above mentioned features, the SmartClip™ Self-Ligating Appliance System has as its basis the MBT™ Versatile+ Appliance System philosophy, which provides orthodontic treatment with low force levels when applying orthodontic mechanics. The general orthodontic principles described in *Systemized Orthodontic Treatment Mechanics* are extensively reviewed in this text to show how these concepts can be used with the SmartClip™ Self-Ligating Appliance. This appliance reduces the friction established between the archwire and the bracket slot, providing good three-dimensional control of the teeth, decreasing treatment time and, at the same time, allowing the clinician to provide excellent treatment results for patients.

Hugo Trevisi

Acknowledgments

It has been three years of hard work since I started this project. The love, care, understanding and companionship of my wife Maria Alice and my children Renata, Rafael and Raquel, have given me the strength to carry on and believe in it. To them, I dedicate my love and care for all these years of being together.

I specially thank Michelle Trevisi de Araujo, who has been with me during all the time of writing this book, working hard to bring quality and success to this project. Thank you.

My sincere acknowledgments to my friends, Dr Richard McLaughlin and Dr John Bennett, working partners for over 30 years. We work together aiming to improve orthodontics.

I would also like to acknowledge many colleagues who dedicated their time and effort to make this project a success: Dr Reginaldo Trevisi Zanelato, Dr Adriano Trevisi Zanelato, Dr André Trevisi Zanelato and Dr Renata C Trevisi from Brazil, Dr Fredrik Bergstrand from Sweden, and Dr Lars Christensen from England. I very much appreciate your hard work and trust. Thanks also to Dr Adilson Hideki Ueno from Brazil.

I acknowledge and very much appreciate the translation work of Michelle Trevisi de Araujo and Teodoro M Lorent from Brazil; and the text revision of the Portuguese co-edition by Maria Olga Orlandi Lasso. I acknowledge the great work of the graphic designers Jorge Lima from Brazil, and Héctor A Santizo from the USA, and the computer systems developer Fernando P Alduino from Brazil. And I also acknowledge and very much appreciate the trust, valuable help and advice given by Michael Parkinson and Barbara Simmons from Elsevier, Edinburgh, and Lotika Singha.

Contents

CHAPTER 1

A historical overview of orthodontic fixed appliances

Introduction

The first attempt to scientifically move a tooth was made in 1728, when a Frenchman, Pierre Fauchard, used an arch-shaped metal band with holes drilled in preselected sites (Fig. 1.1).[1] Malpositioned teeth were tied to the band using thread to achieve the desired tooth movements. Other methods employed by Fauchard included stripping, extraction and luxation of the malpositioned teeth. Pierre Fauchard is considered the father of modern orthodontics.

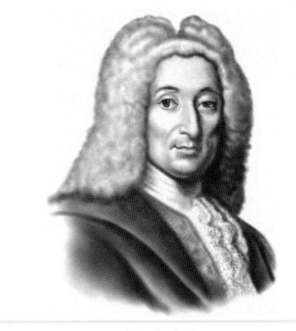

Pierre Fauchard

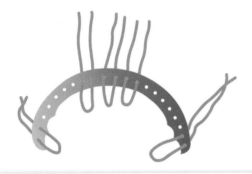

Fig. 1.1 Device invented by Pierre Fauchard to carry out tooth movement.

In about 1860, Norman William Kingsley introduced occipital anchorage. Later, in 1880, he published the 'Treatise on oral deformities as a branch of mechanical surgery', in which he defended dental extractions for some orthodontic cases, which was a controversial issue at that time. Angle considered Kingsley the greatest mastermind of orthodontics.

In 1925, Edward H Angle introduced the Edgewise Appliance, on which modern orthodontic appliances are based.[2] This appliance had identical brackets for all teeth, and tooth movement was accomplished by adding bends to the rectangular archwires. Edgewise appliances continue to be used by many clinicians today.

In 1952, with the aim of decreasing the need for second order bends in orthodontic archwires, Holdaway introduced some angulation to the brackets, thus simplifying the handling of archwires.[3] Holdaway stated that this would assist with root parallelism and control posterior anchorage by distal angulation of teeth. In 1960, Jarabak adopted the angulated brackets recommended by Holdaway and became the first orthodontist to use angulated brackets in two planes of space.[4]

In 1970, Andrews further simplified orthodontic treatment with the introduction of the Straight-Wire™ Appliance, a fully programmed appliance. After Andrews, several orthodontists launched their own bracket prescriptions. Those aimed at simplifying orthodontic treatment, and providing more comfort to patients, have been more successful.

Angle and the birth of orthodontics

Dr Edward Hartley Angle's innovations established him as one of the greatest names in orthodontics and as the professional to give birth to this specialization. Angle was born on June 1, 1855, in Herrick, Pennsylvania. He graduated in orthodontics in 1878 from the Pennsylvania College of Dental Surgery and published his first work in 1887, entitled 'Notes on orthodontics, as a new system for normalization and retention'. In 1889, he wrote an article in which he categorized the types of occlusion on the basis of the mesiodistal relation of the first molars. In the same year, he gave a course at his clinic in St. Louis, Missouri, founding the Angle School of Orthodontics – the first school of orthodontics. In June of the following year, the course was held again and the participants helped found the Society of Orthodontists.

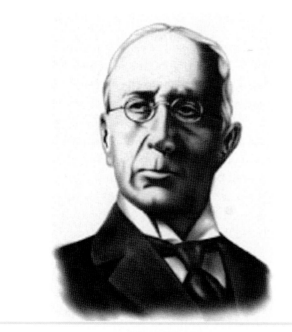

Edward H Angle

Angle believed that orthodontics should be a separate branch of dentistry. Due to his efforts, in 1901 orthodontics became recognized as the first specialty in dentistry. In 1906, Anna Hopkins, newly graduated in orthodontics, became Mrs Edward H Angle. She also joined Angle in the teaching of the new specialty. Enchanted by southern California, the Angles moved to Pasadena in 1916, where, in 1922, with grants provided by former students, they built the Edward H Angle College of Orthodontics in their backyard, the first building erected especially for the teaching of orthodontics. There they gathered some of their followers, such as Spencer Atkinson, Paul Raymond Begg, Cecil Steiner and Allan G Brodie.

In 1890, Angle introduced the E arch. This very simple appliance was capable of providing good alignment of the teeth, and it was the first device to use the molars for fixed anchorage. It required use of bands with buccal tubes on the molars. An expansion archwire was fitted into the buccal tubes and held in place by screws on the tubes. The deficiencies presented by the appliance led Angle to conclude that bodily movement of teeth was needed for more stable results.

To address the need for bodily movement, in 1910 Angle developed the pin and tube appliance, the first appliance to have gold and platinum bands and attachments for most teeth.[5] However, this appliance was difficult to handle and required great skill on the part the clinician. To ensure that the force passed in the right direction through the roots of the teeth, the pins and tubes were assembled parallel to the long axis of the teeth and to each other. In cases where the root needed to be moved more than the crown, the pin had to be welded at an angle that corresponded with the final desired position of the tooth. To keep the appliance activated, it was necessary to keep changing the position of the pins during the treatment. Angle claimed that this was the first mechanism to physiologically control the distribution of forces, and result in movements that were in harmony with the supporting tissues of the tooth. Nevertheless, it was not possible to obtain control of rotation with this appliance.

In 1916, Angle stated that the ideal appliance would be one that could provide light and continuous forces in the desired directions, reduce patient discomfort, and was easy to set up and handle. Hence, because the pin and tube device was difficult to construct, Angle developed the ribbon appliance,[6] a mechanism which included a delicate metal device welded to bands. This device was called a 'bracket' by Angle. In this appliance, the rectangular archwires were passively engaged, with bends added to them, and little by little they would assume an ideal shape, bringing the teeth into the desired positions. Thus, with this appliance, forces began to be transmitted to the teeth through brackets, rather than through other attachments. The archwires were kept in the bracket slot with a closing-pin system which, besides stabilizing the archwires, provided mesiodistal force to the teeth.

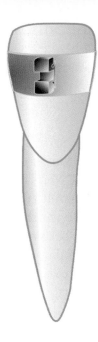

Fig. 1.3   Brackets welded to bands adapted and cemented to the teeth.

Angle: Edgewise Appliance

After several experiments with the appliances described in the previous section, Angle changed the design of the bracket, placing the bracket slot in the center and in the horizontal part of the device, thus increasing the efficiency and precision of the appliance. On June 2, 1925, at a meeting of the Angle Society in Berkeley, California, Angle presented his most important contribution to orthodontics: the Edgewise Appliance[7] (Figs 1.2 & 1.3). This appliance made use of rectangular archwires, which were held in the bracket

slot using metal ligatures.[8] The first brackets were made of gold; however, because of the softness of the gold they tended to lose their shape easily due to the force generated by the occlusion and the metal ligatures. Nevertheless, gold was used because it could be heat treated until it reached satisfactory stiffness, and it was also highly resistant to corrosion. This appliance had a .022/.028 bracket slot.

The Edgewise Appliance allowed movement of the teeth in all directions.[9] With the addition of third order bends, it became possible to move not just the crowns, but the roots as well. Angle advised clinicians to introduce the second order bends in the archwire jointly with the first order bends to improve anchorage control of the posterior teeth and reduce the active treatment time. However, rotation was still difficult to accomplish. So attachments were welded to the mesial and distal of the brackets to help with rotation (Fig. 1.4). The Edgewise Appliance, as originally devised by Angle, was developed for treatment without extractions, where there was no need for space closure mechanics. This appliance supplied the needs of that time.

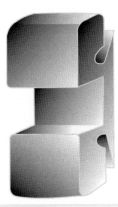

Fig. 1.2   The Edgewise Appliance developed by Angle. Note the slot in the center of the bracket.

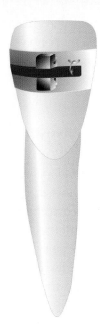

Fig. 1.4 Small hooks were welded to the mesial or distal of the brackets to help correct rotations.

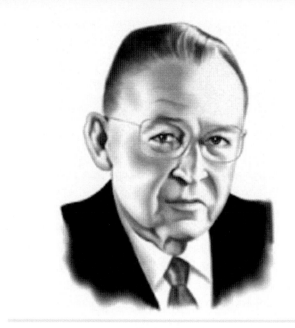

Charles H Tweed

In February 1929, in Arizona, Charles H Tweed, one of Angle's disciples, became the first specialist in orthodontics. Angle died on August 11 of the following year in Santa Monica, California.

I finished my work as perfect as it was possible to do it.
Edward Hartley Angle

Tweed: Edgewise Appliance

Although Angle was the inventor of the Edgewise Appliance, much of the responsibility for testing it and disseminating its philosophy was left to his disciple and friend Charles H Tweed. In 1928, after several months of working with Angle, Tweed established the first clinic specializing in the use of the Edgewise Appliance in Tucson, Arizona.

In 1932, Tweed published his first paper on Angle's principles entitled 'Reports of cases treated with the Edgewise arch mechanism'. Tweed continued to be guided by Angle's 'non-extractionist' philosophy, but gradually he adopted tooth extractions as a way of correcting malocclusions, because some of the cases treated by his colleagues tended to relapse. In 1936, Tweed left the Angle Society and later published his first work on dental extractions. As a result, Tweed came to be considered by Angle's disciples as a traitor to the original edgewise appliance philosophy.

Even at that time, the demand for orthodontic treatment was high, and patients waited for months to receive treatment. This era became known as the 'Golden Age' of orthodontics, although the treatment per se was still quite primitive. Patients spent a long and uncomfortable time in the clinician's chair while the bands were being individually made. In addition, heavy forces were transmitted to the teeth using very stiff and heavy wires, which were kept activated for weeks. Stainless steel brackets and bands gradually replaced the gold brackets and bands. In 1952, Brainerd F Swain[10] developed the twin bracket (Fig. 1.5), which was promptly incorporated into the Edgewise Appliance. Brackets of different sizes started to be used for the different groups of teeth.

Tweed's contribution went beyond just testing the Edgewise Appliance. He developed an entire treatment philosophy with an emphasis on diagnosis, thus popularizing cephalometrics. Tweed's philosophy was concerned with facial esthetics and he developed the concept of uprighting teeth on the basal bone, with an

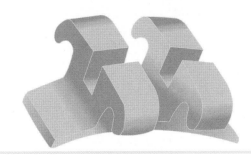

Fig. 1.5 The twin bracket developed by Brainerd F Swain and later incorporated into the Edgewise Appliance.

emphasis on the lower incisors. In addition, besides making extraction of teeth acceptable for orthodontic correction, he introduced the idea of anchorage as an important part of treatment. Many concepts advocated by Tweed became fundamental principles in orthodontics. Tweed's treatment philosophy prevented the Edgewise Appliance from falling into oblivion, and guided clinicians toward successful orthodontic treatment.

In 1955, Levern Merrifield, one of Tweed's most brilliant students, joined his team and made some contributions to the technique that became part of the Tweed teaching courses. Concepts such as tooth size

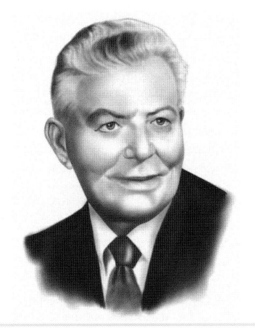

Levern Merrifield

discrepancy and analysis of the lower third of the face started to be followed, contributing to a more precise diagnosis. In addition, Merrifield introduced improvements to the Edgewise Appliance, making it easier to work with.

Tweed–Merrifield: Edgewise Appliance

Merrifield applied Tweed's concepts to develop force systems that simplified the use of the Edgewise Appliance.[11] The precise use of customized archwires was crucial for achieving good results with the Edgewise Appliance. Tweed used up to 12 pairs of customized archwires during treatment. Merrifield reduced the number to five pairs. Basically, the foundation of the Tweed–Merrifield edgewise appliance philosophy consisted of five sequential concepts:

1. Sequential set-up of the appliance, allowing increased comfort and reduced chair time for the patient.
2. Use of customized archwires during the first months of treatment to establish greater inter-bracket distance that in turn provided more elasticity to the wires.
3. Individual or within-group movement of teeth, leading to faster tooth movement.
4. Establishment of mandibular anchorage first, allowing fast preparation of anchorage by tipping two teeth at a time until they reached the desired position. High-pull headgear was used to support the Class III elastics (known as the directional force system, whereby upward and forward force vectors are used to position the teeth vertically in relation to the basal bone).
5. Establishment of vertical control, so that facial esthetics were not compromised.

Begg: Begg Technique

Paul Raymond Begg was born in 1898 in Coolgardie, Australia. In 1924 he moved to Pasadena, California, where he spent two years under Angle's tutoring. Before returning to Australia in 1925, under Angle's supervision, he manufactured the first edgewise bracket using a lathe. Thus he was one of the first clinicians to test the new appliance. Begg published his first work entitled 'Normal occlusion and malocclusion', in the *Australian Journal of Dentistry* in 1926, and this paper marked the beginning of a long career in orthodontics.

Begg reviewed Angle's views on diagnosis and in 1928 he embraced the concept of tooth extractions.[12] In 1930, Begg started using round archwires in his treatments and, in 1933, he launched the Begg technique with Angle's ribbon appliance as a basis, but with the slot guide oriented to the gingival. In the early 1940s, he teamed up with a metal worker, Arthur Wilcock, to design a series of round stainless steel wires with specific stiffness and flexibility, thus making possible the development of his technique. The ribbon

appliance brackets, rotated 180° were used for this technique (Fig. 1.6). Closing pins held the wires in the brackets, allowing the wires to move the teeth in all directions, without compromising tooth movement.[12]

Begg's technique was essentially developed for cases that required extractions and treatment was done with round archwires only. These wires were stiff enough to prevent deformation from the masticatory forces but had sufficient elasticity for the insertion of bends without breaking. Such characteristics allowed application of forces for long periods with small loss of force, thus needing less frequent activation.

One of the main characteristics of this technique was the concept of differential force, in which tooth movement was planned on the basis of anchorage control obtained from the posterior teeth, thus avoiding the use of headgear. Light forces of approximately 65 g were applied to retract the anterior teeth. Forces of this magnitude did not lead to anchorage loss of the posterior teeth,[13] but any increase in force would lead to the loss of posterior anchorage and, consequently, no distalization of the anterior teeth.

After dedicating most of his life time to orthodontics, Begg died on January 18, 1983.

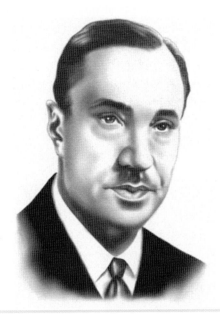

Paul R Begg

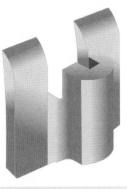

Fig. 1.6   The Begg bracket with vertical slot.

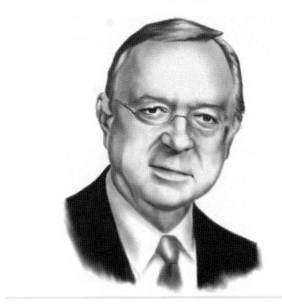

Lawrence F Andrews

Andrews: Straight-Wire™ Technique

The Edgewise Appliance requires incorporating bends in the rectangular archwires in the three planes of space to obtain an ideal occlusion.

In 1970, Lawrence F Andrews, in an attempt to eliminate the need for archwire bends, developed the Straight-Wire™ Appliance. The concept behind this appliance was that the brackets would move the teeth in the desired direction.[14] Andrews' concept was based on his research involving measurement of 120 cases with normal natural occlusion. The aim of this study was to determine the positioning and the size of each tooth in the dental arch. On the basis of his results, Andrews designed a bracket system that had in its prescription angulation, inclination and in–out. However, orthodontic treatment with this appliance was based on the similarities in the morphology of naturally occurring normal occlusions. All or almost all of the entire treatment was carried out without archwire bending,[15] except when bends were needed for detailing and in situations outside normality.

Although the Straight-Wire™ Appliance was another innovation, the heavy forces of the edgewise technique continued to be part of the treatment mechanics. In its early years, numerous biomechanical problems were encountered due to the excess force and possibly due to the extra angulation built in the brackets for the anterior teeth. Deepening of overbite, protrusion and lateral open bite – known as the 'roller coaster effect' – occurred in many cases.

Before launching the Straight-Wire™ Appliance, Andrews drew attention to the 'wagon wheel effect', that is, loss of angulation as torque was added. So he incorporated extra angulation into the brackets for the anterior teeth (Fig. 1.7). Andrews also believed that the center of the clinical crown was easy to visualize by clinicians, and thus this became the reference point for positioning the brackets.

The Straight-Wire™ appliance was initially developed for cases without extractions. However, it also started to be used for extraction cases, which required rotational control and increased bracket angulation. To further improve the appliance, Andrews developed a series of Straight-Wire™ brackets for extraction cases, incorporating the concepts of angulation, torque and first order bends. He also introduced three different specifications of torque for the upper and lower incisors, cross-referencing their application with the ANB angle of each patient. Thus the appliance became available in several prescriptions.

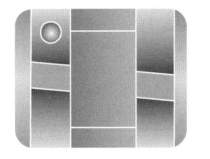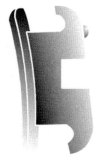

Fig. 1.7   Straight-Wire™ bracket: square-shaped with torque in the base.

From observations on the same 120 models that formed the basis of new appliance, Andrews noted the presence of six consistent, recurring characteristics. As significant as the development of Straight-Wire™ Appliance, these characteristics were classified and presented by him in a paper published in 1972, entitled 'Six keys to normal occlusion'. The six characteristics are:[16]

● Inter-arch relationship
● Crown angulation
● Crown inclination
● Lack of rotation
● Tight contact points
● Curve of Spee.

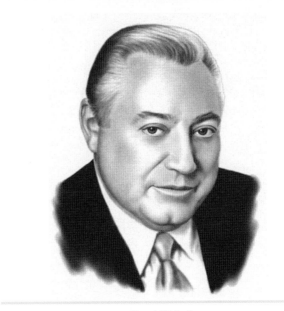

Ronald H Roth

These characteristics are very important for clinicians to keep in mind when treating their patients.

Roth: Straight-Wire™ Technique

The Straight-Wire™ Appliance became widely accepted, and one of the orthodontists who collaborated in its evolution was Ronald H Roth. On the basis of his initial experience with the Straight-Wire™ Appliance, Roth verified that the appliance had many advantages, helping to establish a good functional occlusion and providing good orthodontic results. However, in 1975, he modified the original prescription to solve the problems he faced in his daily clinical application of the appliance. Andrews, in the first generation of the preadjusted appliance, recommended a large range of bracket specifications, but Roth tried to avoid the difficulties associated with a complicated multiple bracket inventory. He recommended the use of a single appliance system that consisted of a minimum number of brackets which, according to him, would allow management of both extraction and non-extraction cases. So Roth introduced a major change to the original prescription of the Straight-Wire™ Appliance, and this system became the 'second generation' preadjusted appliance. Roth's recommendations were received with great enthusiasm because other clinicians had also experienced similar problems with the treatment mechanics, and some were puzzled by Andrews' variety of brackets.[17]

In addition, when analyzing orthodontic results with cast models precisely transferred to articulators, Roth identified functional problems, even in cases that seemed to have been treated successfully. He showed that these discrepancies were not evident when simply observing the models, but could be detected clinically or when casts were mounted on an articulator. Consequently, Roth's approach came to be based on the use of articulators to confirm the diagnosis and to construct splints for jaw repositioning. This approach was used to help establish the correct condyle position. As advocated by Andrews, Roth also used the center of the clinical crown for bracket positioning. He used wider arch forms to improve the inclination of the canines and to achieve better function during lateroprotrusive movements.

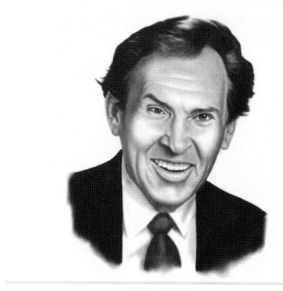

Robert M Ricketts

Ricketts: Bioprogressive™ Technique

In 1976, Robert Murray Ricketts proposed a change in the edgewise technique to make it more flexible and versatile, and introduced the Bioprogressive™ Technique.[18] Ricketts' changes were based on studies conducted on skulls with normal occlusion, and were also drawn from clinical experience. The prefix 'Bio' was adopted to emphasize the close relationship of the technique with biology, involving an overall treatment concept rather than just mechanical and technical sequential steps. The biological concepts of growth, development and function were applied in a manner that would help normalize the physiology and improve esthetics. The term 'Progressive' was used to express the treatment sequence.

In the standard Bioprogressive™ Technique, torque and inclination are incorporated in some brackets and buccal tubes, with the aim of positioning the teeth without the need to add bends to the wires. When Ricketts presented his prescription he stated that the 22° torque for the upper central incisor could seem excessive; however, the torque could only be fully expressed if rectangular or square archwires were used throughout the treatment. Ricketts recommended overcorrection in patients with Class II division 2 malocclusion or with interincisal angles of 125° or less. For the upper lateral incisor, he initially recommended torque of 17° and angulation of 5°; later, based on further experience, the prescription was changed to 14° torque and 8° angulation.

For the lower posterior segment, Ricketts recommended progressive torque, to the extent that the first premolar would be vertically positioned in relation to the occlusal plane and the second premolar crowns would be positioned more toward the lingual. His research indicated that lower first molars had between 20° and 25° torque, and he recommended 22° torque for these teeth. For the second molars, the recommendation was 0°. Ricketts also considered that the torque of the lower molar roots was very important to obtain adequate anchorage when using the Bioprogressive™ Technique.

Toward the end of the 1980s, Ricketts and Gugino introduced changes to the Bioprogressive™ Technique and developed three sets of brackets: one set for brachyfacial individuals, one for mesofacial, and one for dolichofacial individuals, because each group has typically shaped dental arches. These new sets of brackets were denominated proversion, neutroversion and retroversion brackets, respectively.

The proversion brackets were indicated for use mainly in patients with deep bite and Class II division 2 malocclusion, and for some Class II division 1 malocclusions. The neutroversion brackets were indicated for Class I cases with moderate anterior open bite or deep bite. The retroversion brackets were indicated for uprighting the upper incisors. They were also indicated for Class II division 1 patients who needed to wear elastics.

Nowadays, the device most widely known from the Bioprogressive™ Technique is the utility arch.[19] This archwire is manufactured from .016/.016 blue Elgiloy and can be used right from the beginning of treatment. It allows intraoral adjustments, with application of light and continuous forces and torque control. Vertical discrepancies are treated prior to horizontal discrepancies.

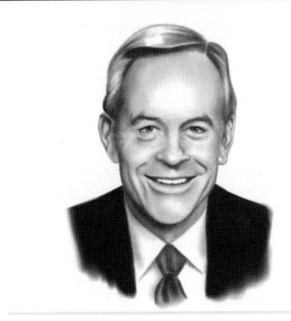

Wick R G Alexander

Alexander: Vari Simplex Discipline

With the aim of achieving good orthodontic results in the easiest and most efficient way and providing comfort for the patient during treatment, in 1978 Wick Alexander proposed a new treatment philosophy named the Vari Simplex Discipline. The term 'Vari' refers to the range of brackets used and 'Simplex' to the principle 'Keep it simple, Sir!'.

In the Vari Simplex technique, archwires with welded hooks and bends were rarely used, because besides taking time to construct, they encourage accumulation of food and are detrimental to gingival health. When hooks were necessary, they were added to the brackets.[20] Uprighting of lower first molars and lower incisors, which was part of Tweed's philosophy, was also a part of the technique. With the aim of decreasing the number of bends added to the archwires and improving the orthodontic results, Alexander incorporated a 6° angulation on the tubes of the lower first molars in his prescription. To obtain a more upright positioning of the lower incisors, centralizing their roots in the basal bone, −5° torque was added to the brackets of these teeth, thus preventing their buccal inclination. Twin and single-wing preadjusted brackets were used concurrently. These different types of bracket had a .018 slot and were used according to the needs of each tooth. Characteristics such as shape, size, mesiodistal length and curvature of the teeth affect the inter-bracket distance and interfere with the aligning and leveling of the teeth. As well as this, according to Alexander, patient comfort needed to be considered when choosing the brackets. Twin brackets were used for teeth with large and flat surfaces, such as the upper incisors. For the posterior teeth single-wing brackets were preferred. The increased inter-bracket distance allowed the use of multistrand rectangular wires at the beginning of treatment. Fewer wires were needed, and .017/.025 flexible rectangular archwires were engaged in the brackets early in the treatment, allowing adequate torque control during the entire treatment.

Thus, with esthetics as his main goal, Alexander was convinced that a good orthodontic result was based on an esthetically pleasant face associated with stability of treatment and a balanced occlusion.

McLaughlin, Bennett and Trevisi: MBT™ Versatile+ Appliance System

With the aim of overcoming the inadequacies of the original Straight-Wire™ Appliance, McLaughlin, Bennett and Trevisi combined their efforts to design a new system of brackets.[21] They reviewed Andrews' original findings and took into account additional research from Japan.[22,23] On the basis of their findings, and many years of clinical experience, they designed the MBT™ Appliance System, which was officially introduced in 1997. This third generation preadjusted bracket system has retained all that was best in the original design, but at the same time has introduced a range of improvements to the specifications to help solve clinical problems.

The MBT™ Appliance[21] was designed to work with sliding mechanics, whereby light, continuous forces are applied. The rectangular brackets were replaced by rhomboidal brackets (Fig. 1.8). This change reduced the bulk of each bracket and coordinated perspective lines through only two planes so that bracket positioning became more precise. This innovative bracket system has versatility, that is, it can be applied in most clinical situations, avoids insertion of bends in the archwires and also helps in inventory control.[21]

The excessive angulation for the anterior teeth in Andrews' and Roth's prescriptions was a great disadvantage because it led to loss of anterior anchorage, and a tendency for bite deepening during leveling and aligning. In some cases, the root of the

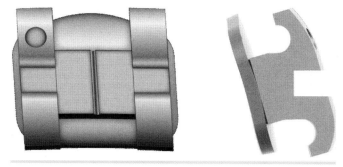

Fig. 1.8   MBT™ bracket: rhomboid-shaped with torque in base.

upper canine was placed very near the root of the first premolar. In the MBT™ Appliance System, the angulation for the anterior brackets is based on the values obtained by Andrews in his study (Fig. 1.9). Consequently, the tendency for deep bite is reduced and anchorage control increased, requiring less cooperation from the patient.

The MBT™ Appliance System has additional positive torque for the upper incisors, additional negative torque for the upper molars, additional negative torque for the lower incisors and reduced negative torque from the canines to the lower second molars.[21] These alterations have been significant in meeting the clinical objectives of treatment and reducing the need for wire bending (Fig. 1.10).

Typical orthodontic cases are different from the 120 non-extraction adult cases studied by Andrews. Hence it was decided that three torque options are necessary for the canines, and the MBT™ Appliance System brackets for the upper canines can have −7°, 0° or +7° torque, which ensures versatility of the appliance. Similarly, the brackets for the lower canines are available with −6°, 0° and +6° torque. Following some of the principles advocated by Andrews, a bracket positioning system and a chart for guiding the positioning of the brackets were also developed. This technique allows better precision in the vertical positioning of brackets.

The MBT™ Appliance System was developed to overcome the challenges faced in most treatments and displays a series of innovations in comparison with other appliances developed in the past. There are seven different possibilities of using brackets and buccal tubes, depending on the need of each case (Fig.1.11). This establishes a platform that allows the bracket system to be individualized and achieve the overcorrection required in some cases.

In summary, the MBT™ Appliance System emerged from the need to design brackets for sliding mechanics with light forces, and to meet modern concepts of bracket design and versatility.

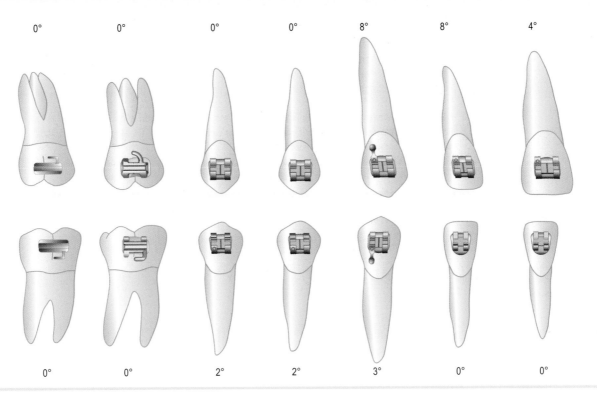

Fig. 1.9   MBT™ Appliance: bracket angulation.

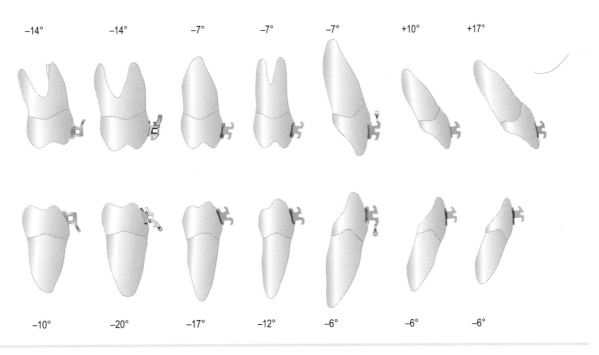

Fig. 1.10   MBT™ Appliance: bracket torque.

Versatility options presented by the appliance
1. 180° bracket rotation for the upper lateral incisor in cases of crossbite, providing −10° torque
2. Three torque options for the upper canines (−7°, 0° and +7°)
3. Three torque options for the lower canines (−6°, 0° and +6°)
4. Using the tubes of the lower second and first molars on the upper first and second molars from the opposite side in cases finishing with a Class II molar relationship
5. 180° bracket rotation for the upper canine in cases with agenesis of the upper lateral incisor when the treatment plan is to close space
6. Interchangeable brackets for the upper premolars – same angulation and torque
7. Interchangeable brackets for the lower incisors – same angulation and torque

Fig. 1.11   Versatility options: the MBT™ Appliance System.

SmartClip™ Self-Ligating Appliance System

The SmartClip™ Self-Ligating Appliance System is more than just another bracket prescription, because it is a new appliance concept, applying low forces and reducing friction. This system presents an advance in bracket design, and has revolutionized the method of engagement and disengagement of archwires.

The SmartClip™ brackets self-ligating mechanism consists of two Nitinol clips that open and close automatically through elastic deformation of the material when the archwire exerts a force on the clips (Fig. 1.12). The clips allow easy engagement and disengagement of the archwires in the bracket slot.[24] Such a feature allows optimal forces to be applied during the entire treatment, promoting more efficient and physiological tooth movement, and therefore is more comfortable for the patient.

The reduction of the classic problem of friction with the SmartClip™ self-ligating bracket allows the archwire to work freely within the bracket slot, thus improving the efficiency of the sliding mechanics. Thus time spent on the aligning, leveling and space closure is reduced. In addition, patient chair time is reduced, because of the ease of engagement and disengagement of the archwires, which in some cases can be engaged in the bracket slot using just the fingers. Elimination of elastic ligatures also helps improve the patient's oral hygiene.

The SmartClip™ Self-Ligating Appliance System design follows the MBT™ Versatile+ Appliance philosophy[21] and has additional negative torque for the upper second molar. This provides further versatility to the brackets, control of tooth movements and achievement of the functional occlusion at the end of treatment. In addition, the brackets are available with the APC Plus™ Color Change adhesive, which helps bracket positioning and flash removal. The combination of these factors ensures the efficiency of the SmartClip™ Self-Ligating Appliance and provides excellent treatment results.

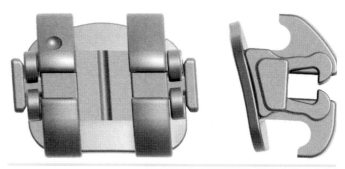

Fig. 1.12   SmartClip™ Self-Ligating Appliance bracket: rhomboidal shaped with torque in base and Nitinol clips.

References

1. Angle E H 1911 Evolution of orthodontics – recent developments. Dental Cosmos 54:853–867

2. Matasa C G, Graber T M 2000 Angle, the innovator, mechanical genius, and clinician. American Journal of Orthodontics 117:444–452

3. Holdaway R A 1952 Bracket angulation as applied to the edgewise appliance. Angle Orthodontist 22:227–236

4. Jarabak J R 1960 Development of a treatment plan in the light of one's concept of treatment objectives. American Journal of Orthodontics and Dentofacial Orthopedics 46:481–514

5. Angle E H 1970 The malocclusion of the teeth. SS White Dental Manufacturing

6. Angle E H 1916 Some new forms of orthodontic mechanism, and the reasons for their introduction. Dental Cosmos 58:969–996

7. Angle E H c1925 Announcement of the Angle College of Orthodontia. Pasadena, California

8. Angle E H 1928 The latest and best in orthodontic mechanism. Dental Cosmos 70:1143–1158

9. Angle E H 1929 The latest and best in orthodontic mechanism. Dental Cosmos 71:260–270

10. Swain B F 1952 Clinical demonstration of the Bull technique. Charles H. Tweed Foundation meeting

11. Vaden J L, Dale J G, Klontz H A 1996 The Edgewise appliance of Tweed–Merrifield: philosophy, diagnosis and treatment. In: Graber T M, Vanarsdall R L (eds). Orthodontics: principles and current techniques, 2nd edn. Guanabara Koogan, Rio de Janeiro, pp 579–635

12. Begg P R, Kesling P C 1971 Begg orthodontic theory and technique, 2nd edn. W B Saunders, Philadelphia

13. Begg P R 1968 The origin and progress of the light wire differential force technique. Begg Journal of Orthodontic Theory and Treatment 4:9–34

14. Andrews L F 1975 The straight-wire appliance: syllabus of philosophy and technique, 2nd edn. San Diego, pp 137–162

15. Andrews L F 1989 Straight-Wire: the concept and appliance. L A Wells, San Diego, p 407

16. Andrews L F 1972 The six keys to normal occlusion. American Journal of Orthodontics 62:296–309

17. Roth R H 1996 Mecânica do tratamento para aparelho straight-wire. In: Graber T M, Vanarsdall R L (eds). Ortodontia: princípios e técnicas atuais, 2nd edn. Guanabara Koogan, Rio de Janeiro, pp 636–660

18. Ricketts R M 1976 Bioprogressive therapy as an answer to orthodontics needs Part I. American Journal of Orthodontics 70:241–268

19. Ricketts R M 1976 Bioprogressive therapy as an answer to orthodontics needs Part II. American Journal of Orthodontics 70:359–397

20. Alexander R G W 1996 The Alexander discipline: contemporary concepts and philosophies. Ormco, Glendora, p 461

21. McLaughlin R P, Bennett J C, Trevisi H J 2001 Systemized orthodontic treatment mechanics. Mosby, Edinburgh, p 342

22. Watanabe K, Koga M, Yatabe K, Motegi E, Isshiki Y A 1996 A morphometric study on setup models of Japanese malocclusions. Shikwa Gakuho 96:209–222

23. Sebata E 1980 An orthodontic study of teeth and dental arch form on the Japanese normal occlusion. Shikwa Gakuho 80:945–969

24. Trevisi H J 2005 The SmartClip™ self-ligating appliance system. Technique Guide. 3M Company

Chapter 1 Clinical Case

Name: B A
Sex: Female
Age: 12.6 years
Facial pattern: Dolichofacial
Skeletal pattern: Class I

Diagnosis

A Class II malocclusion, with crowding in the upper and lower arches, and slightly buccal eruption of the upper canines and the lower left first premolar, irregular incisal edges of the upper incisors, and anatomical abnormality of the upper left canine.

Treatment plan

Extraction of the upper first premolars and lower second premolars with the objective of achieving an occlusion with Class I molar relationship. Use of Class II elastics and reduction of inclination of the lower incisors to maintain a good facial profile.

Appliance

- SmartClip™ self-ligating appliance
- Upper modified Hawley wraparound retainer
- Lower 3–3 fixed retainer

Case report

The patient presented with moderate crowding in the upper and lower arches. First, the upper premolars were extracted and the incisal edges of the upper incisors and the labial surface of the upper left canine were leveled to ensure adequate bracket placement using the indirect bonding technique. Buccal minitubes were bonded to the second premolars. Next the lower second premolars were extracted and the appliance was bonded using the indirect bonding technique.

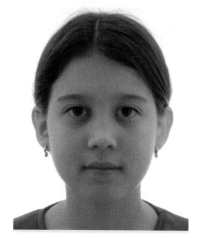 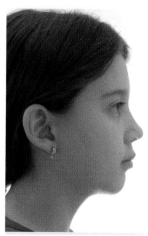

Fig. 1.13   Fig. 1.14

Figs 1.13 & 1.14
Pretreatment photographs showing facial symmetry, Class I facial (skeletal) profile and good lip seal.

.014 and .016 round Nitinol archwires were used during the initial stage of treatment, whereas .018 and .020 round stainless steel archwires were used for leveling. Buccal tubes were bonded to the lower second molars to level the curve of Spee.

During the space closure stage, .019/.025 stainless steel archwires with prewelded hooks mesial to the canines were used, as well as Class II elastics to maintain the Class I molar relationship. In the final stage of treatment, some rebonding was carried out and a .019/.025 rectangular Nitinol archwire was used for re-leveling and a .019/.025 braided archwire for settling of the occlusion.

After fixed appliance removal, a modified Hawley wraparound retainer was fitted in the upper arch and a 3–3 fixed retainer was placed in the lower arch.

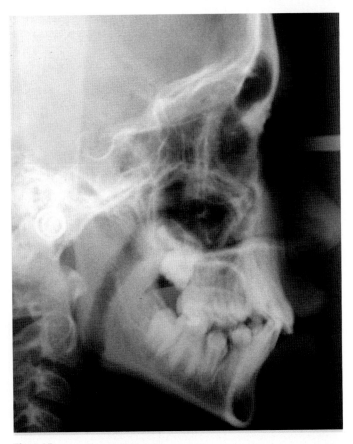

Fig. 1.15

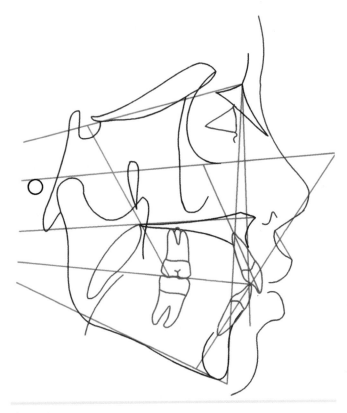

Fig. 1.16

SNA ∠	77°
SNB ∠	73°
ANB ∠	4°
A-N ⊥ FH	−2 mm
Po-N ⊥ FH	−14 mm
Wits	2.8 mm
GoGn SN ∠	38°
FH Md ∠	30°
Mx Md ∠	28°
U1 to A-Po	9 mm
L1 to A-Po	4.5 mm
U1 to Mx plane ∠	111°
L1 to Md plane ∠	98°
Facial analysis	
Nasolabial ∠	92°
NA ⊥ nose	25 mm
Lip thickness	12 mm

Figs 1.15, 1.16 & 1.17
Cephalometric X-ray, tracing and measurements showing moderate protrusion and inclination of the upper and lower incisors.

Fig. 1.17

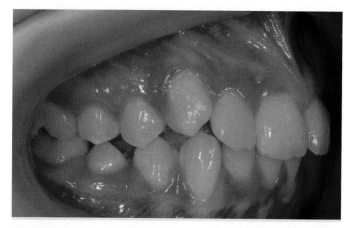

Fig. 1.18

Figs 1.18, 1.19 & 1.20
Pretreatment intraoral photographs showing the Class
II molar relationship with upper and lower crowding
and slightly buccal eruption of the upper canines.

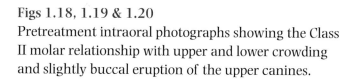

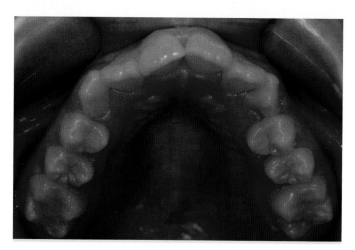

Fig. 1.21

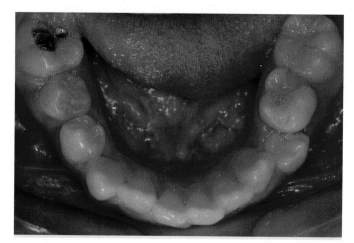

Figs 1.21 & 1.22
Pretreatment upper and lower occlusal views showing
upper and lower anterior crowding and moderate
posterior crowding on the lower left side.

Fig. 1.22

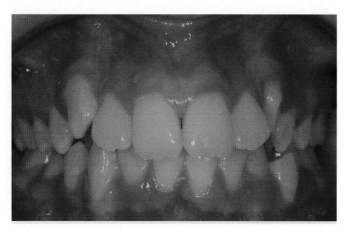

Fig. 1.19

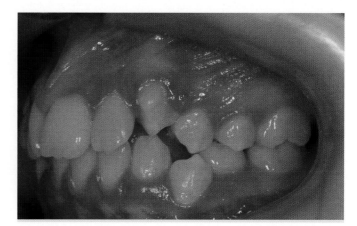

Fig. 1.20

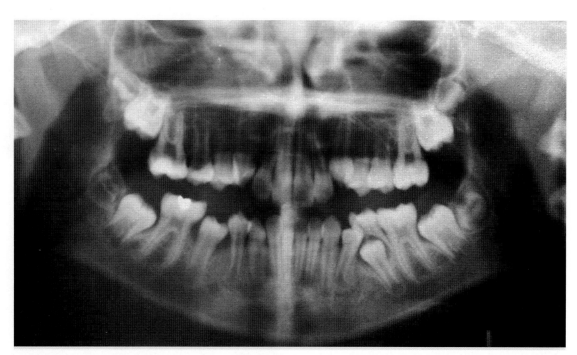

Fig. 1.23

Fig. 1.23
Panoramic X-ray showing some irregularities in the shape of the roots, with lack of space for the lower left second premolar and the lower second molars.

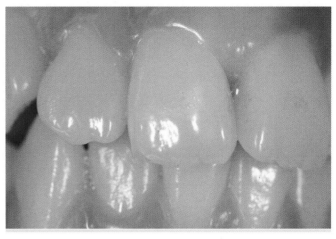

Fig. 1.24

Figs 1.24, 1.25 & 1.26
The irregular incisal edges of the upper incisors, ready for indirect bonding after leveling.

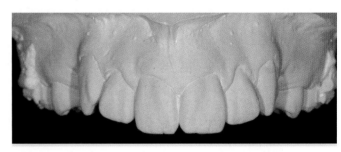

Fig. 1.27

Figs 1.27, 1.28 & 1.29
Study model showing leveling of the incisal edges. Brackets placed on the study model, and silicone tray with brackets ready to be bonded to the patient's teeth.

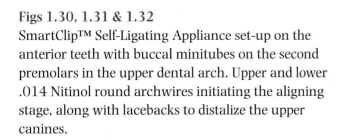

Figs 1.30, 1.31 & 1.32
SmartClip™ Self-Ligating Appliance set-up on the anterior teeth with buccal minitubes on the second premolars in the upper dental arch. Upper and lower .014 Nitinol round archwires initiating the aligning stage, along with lacebacks to distalize the upper canines.

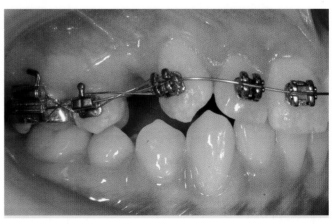

Fig. 1.30

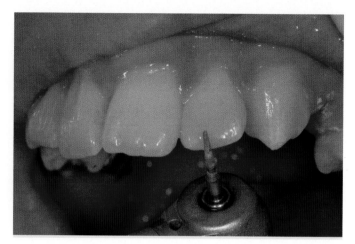

Fig. 1.25

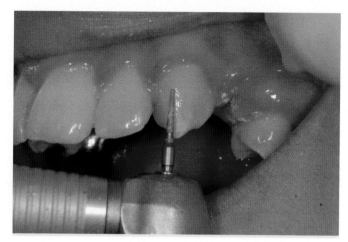

Fig. 1.26

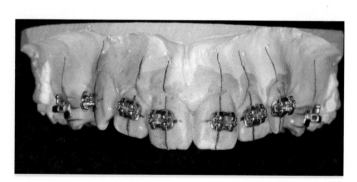

Fig. 1.28

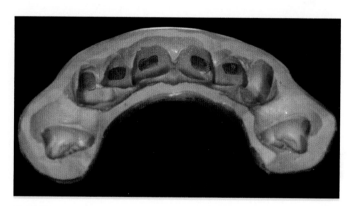

Fig. 1.29

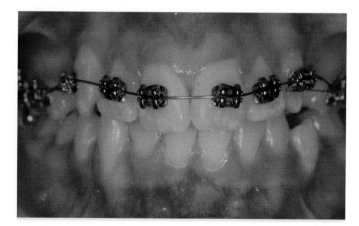

Fig. 1.31

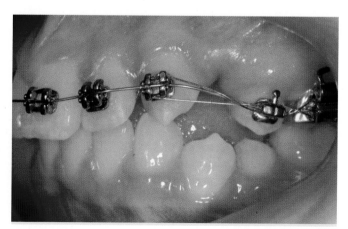

Fig. 1.32

Figs 1.33, 1.34 & 1.35
SmartClip™ Self-Ligating Appliance set-up in both arches with .018 steel round archwire in the upper arch and .016 Nitinol for finalizing leveling in the lower arch. Note the buccal tubes on the lower second molars.

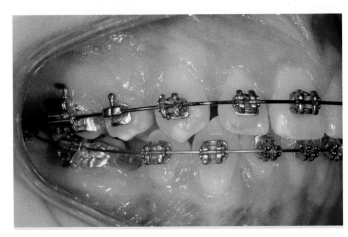

Figs 1.33

Figs 1.36 & 1.37
Upper and lower occlusal views showing .018 steel round archwire in the upper arch and .016 round Nitinol archwire in the lower arch for finalizing leveling. Buccal tubes were placed on the lower second molars to assist in leveling the curve of Spee.

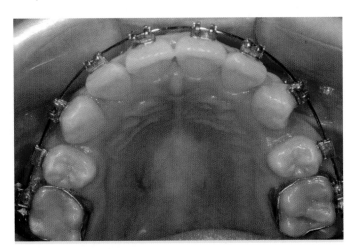

Fig 1.36

Figs 1.38, 1.39 & 1.40
A .018 round Nitinol archwire in the upper arch and .019/.025 stainless steel rectangular archwire in the lower arch to close the residual spaces in the extraction sites. In the upper arch, there was no need for space closure mechanics.

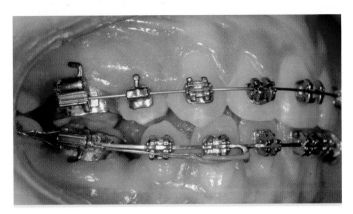

Fig. 1.38

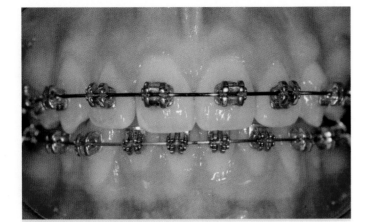

Fig. 1.34

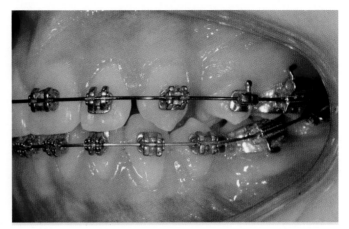

Fig. 1.35

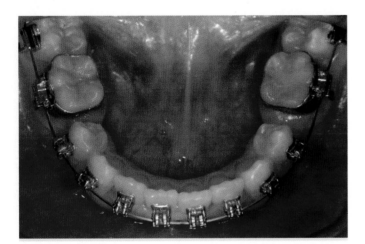

Fig. 1.37

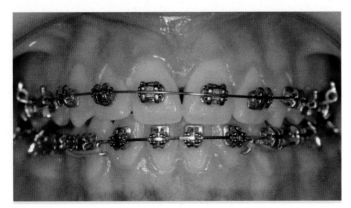

Fig. 1.39

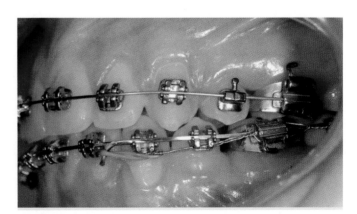

Fig. 1.40

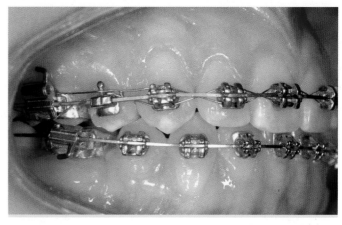

Fig. 1.41

Figs 1.41, 1.42 & 1.43
Upper and lower .019/.025 rectangular Nitinol
archwires for re-leveling after bracket repositioning.

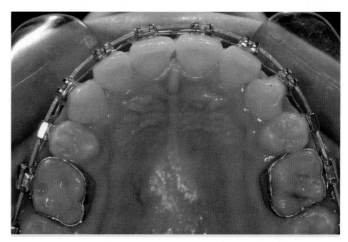

Fig. 1.44

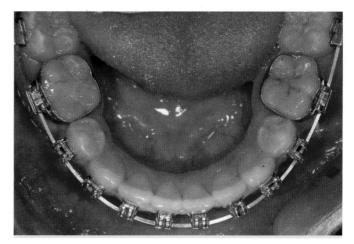

Figs 1.44 & 1.45

Upper and lower occlusal views of .019/.025
rectangular Nitinol archwires in the upper and lower
arches.

Fig. 1.45

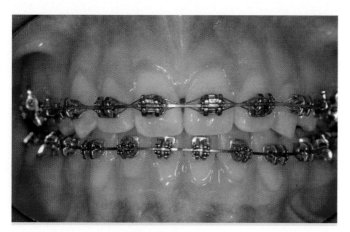

Fig. 1.42

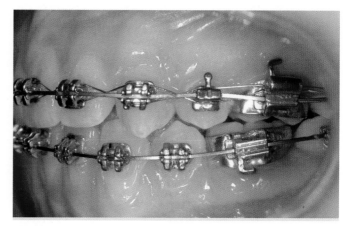

Fig. 1.43

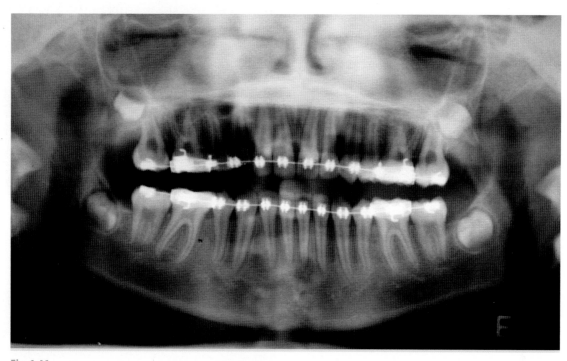

Fig. 1.46

Fig. 1.46
Panoramic X-ray showing root parallelism with some irregularities in root shape.

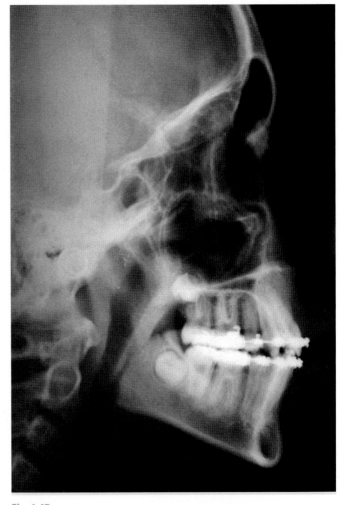

Figs 1.47, 1.48 & 1.49
Interim cephalometric X-ray, tracing and measurements showing reduction of the inclination of the lower incisors.

Fig. 1.47

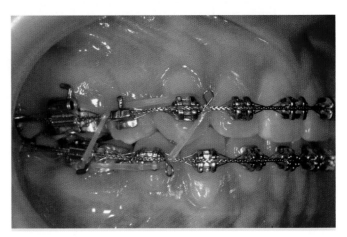

Figs 1.50, 1.51 & 1.52
The final stage of treatment with .019/.025 rectangular braided archwires for settling the occlusion. Note the use of metal ligatures under the brackets to maintain space closure.

Fig. 1.50

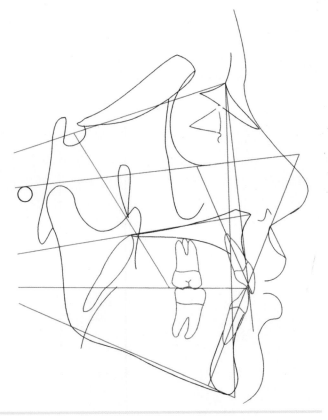

Fig. 1.48

SNA ∠	78°
SNB ∠	74°
ANB ∠	4°
A-N ⊥ FH	0 mm
Po-N ⊥ FH	−8 mm
Wits	3 mm
GoGn SN ∠	39°
FH Md ∠	30°
Mx Md ∠	32°
U1 to A-Po	5 mm
L1 to A-Po	2 mm
U1 to Mx plane ∠	105°
L1 to Md plane ∠	89°
Facial analysis	
Nasolabial ∠	95°
NA ⊥ nose	28 mm
Lip thickness	12 mm

Fig. 1.49

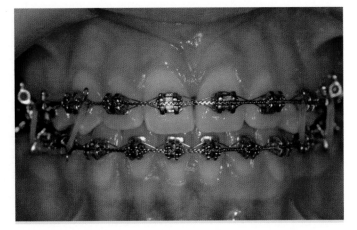

Fig. 1.51

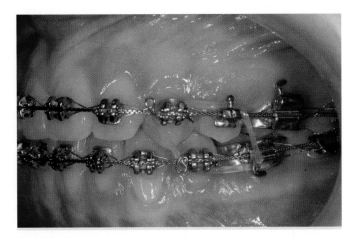

Fig. 1.52

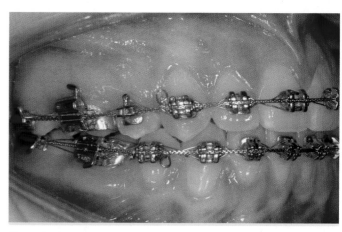

Fig. 1.53

Figs 1.53, 1.54 & 1.55
Upper and lower .019/.025 rectangular braided
archwires after achieving intercuspation.

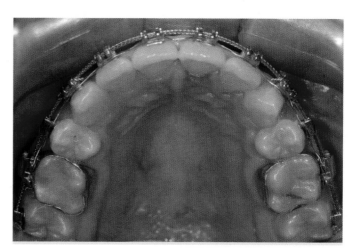

Fig. 1.56

Figs 1.56 & 1.57
Occlusal view with .019/.025 rectangular braided
archwires in the upper and lower arches. There is good
alignment, adequate arch form and the molars are well
positioned.

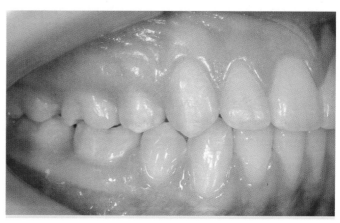

Fig. 1.58

Figs 1.58, 1.59 & 1.60
Post-treatment photographs showing Class I molar and
canine relationships. Upper and lower midlines are
coincident with good overbite for the incisors and the
canines.

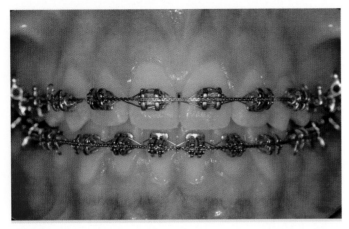

Fig. 1.54

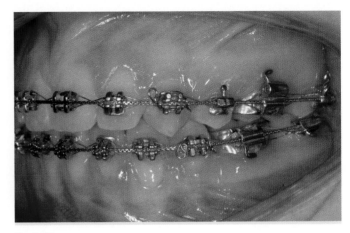

Fig. 1.55

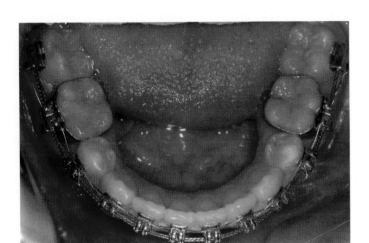

Fig. 1.57

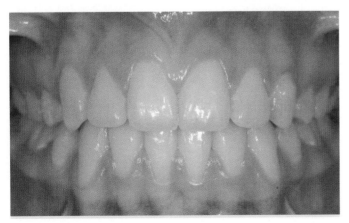

Fig. 1.59

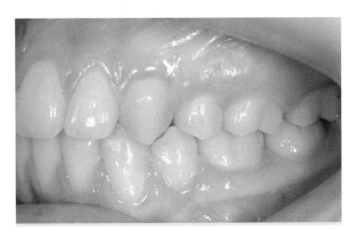

Fig. 1.60

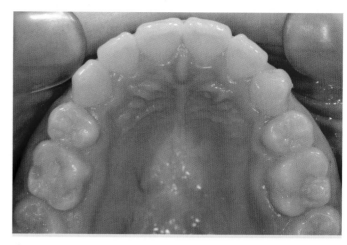

Fig. 1.61

Figs 1.61 & 1.62
Post-treatment upper and lower occlusal views showing the dental arch forms and the positioning of the molars.

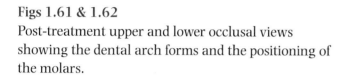

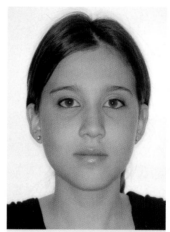

Figs 1.63 & 1.64
Post-treatment facial photographs: frontal and lateral views showing facial symmetry and good facial profile.

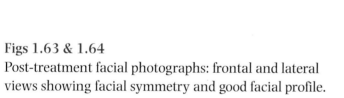

Fig. 1.63   Fig. 1.64

Figs 1.65 & 1.66
Post-treatment facial three-quarter view photographs showing a good smile line.

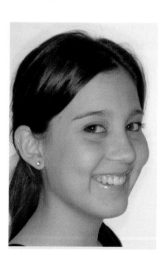

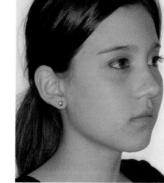

Fig. 1.65   Fig. 1.66

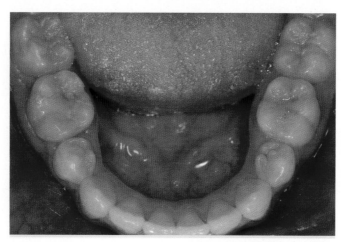

Fig. 1.62

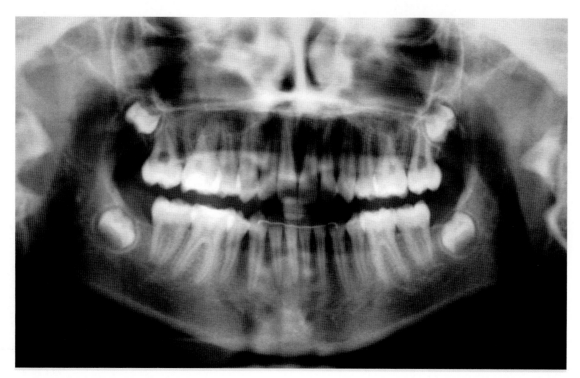

Fig. 1.67

Fig. 1.67
Post-treatment panoramic X-ray showing root parallelism.

Figs 1.68, 1.69, 1.70 & 1.71
Final cephalometric X-ray, tracing and measurements
showing well positioned incisors. Superimposition
shows good control of the vertical growth

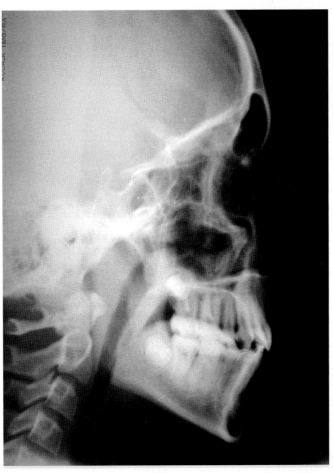

Fig. 1.68

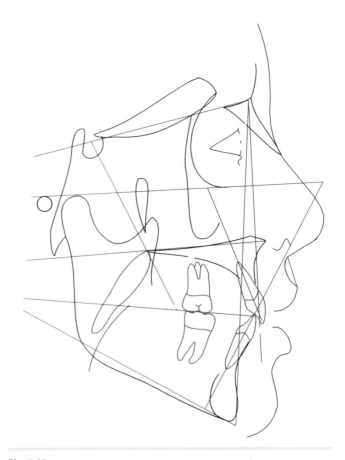

Fig. 1.69

SNA ∠	78°
SNB ∠	74°
ANB ∠	4°
A-N ⊥ FH	0.5 mm
Po-N ⊥ FH	–9 mm
Wits	3 mm
GoGn SN ∠	40°
FH Md ∠	30°
Mx Md ∠	32°
U1 to A-Po	5 mm
L1 to A-Po	2 mm
U1 to Mx plane ∠	109°
L1 to Md plane ∠	90°

Facial analysis

Nasolabial ∠	101°
NA ⊥ nose	28 mm
Lip thickness	12 mm

Fig. 1.70

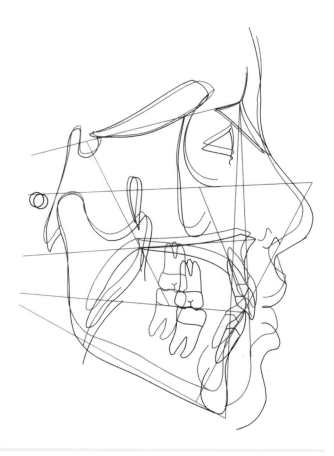

Fig. 1.71

Development of the SmartClip™ Self-Ligating Appliance System

Introduction

The SmartClip™ Self-Ligating Appliance System design follows the MBT™ Versatile+ system philosophy in terms of maximum versatility, mid-size twin brackets, bracket prescription and the use of light forces.[1] The SmartClip™ Self-Ligating Appliance System is classified as a 'passive' bracket system because the archwire works freely within the bracket slot, without any pressure from the clip onto the orthodontic archwire.

The SmartClip™ bracket's self-ligating mechanism consists of two Nitinol clips that open and close automatically through elastic deformation of the material when the archwire exerts a force on the clip.[2] Hand instruments are available to make the engagement and disengagement of archwires easier.

The SmartClip™ Self-Ligating Appliance System consists of three parts:

1. Mesh bonding base
2. The bracket body
3. A pair of clips (Fig. 2.1).

The main bracket body is manufactured using the metal injection molding process. A high-precision laser cuts the Nitinol clip, which is then smoothened. The bracket and the clip are held together by mechanical means and the mesh bonding base is laser-welded onto the bracket body base. The SmartClip™ self-ligating brackets also have the same features as the conventional twin brackets, which allows the use of elastic ligatures, metal ligatures, elastic chain, elastics and all other accessories used with conventional techniques.

Nitinol clip design

Each bracket has a pair of clips made of Nitinol. Careful engineering of the geometry of the clip ensures appropriate force levels during archwire engagement and disengagement and stress–strain distribution for fatigue resistance. Finite element analysis (FEA) computer simulation software was used to predict the forces and stress–strain distribution during archwire engagement and disengagement. In addition, extensive laboratory testing was done to verify the results of the FEA (Figs 2.2, 2.3, 2.4, 2.5, 2.6 & 2.7).

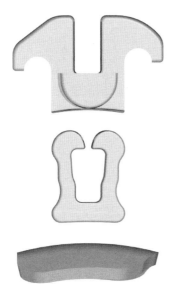

Fig. 2.1 Parts of the SmartClip™ self-ligating bracket: mesh bonding base, Nitinol clip and bracket body.

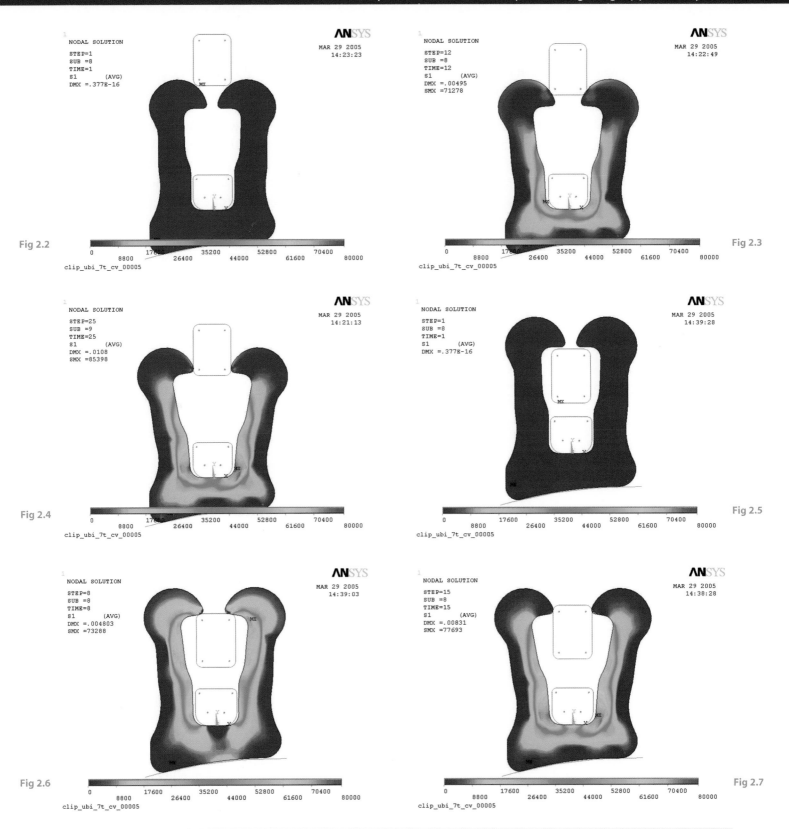

Figs 2.2, 2.3, 2.4, 2.5, 2.6 & 2.7 Finite element analysis of the force and stress–strain distribution in the Nitinol clip during engagement and disengagement of the .019/.025 archwire.

Figures 2.8 and 2.9 show that the stresses induced in the clip during archwire engagement and disengagement are less than the ultimate strength of Nitinol, thus ensuring adequate fatigue life. The forces needed to engage and disengage a .019/.025 rectangular archwire are about 13 N and 20 N, respectively, and correspondingly less for smaller wires.

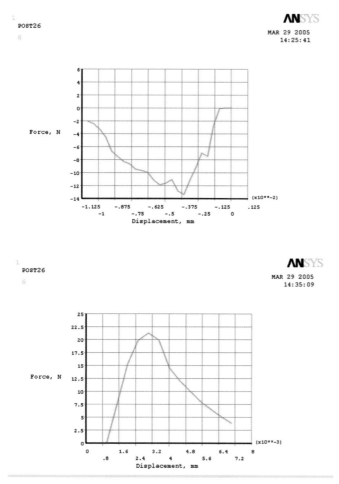

Figs 2.8 & 2.9 Stresses in the clip during engagement and disengagement of a .019/.025 archwire.

SmartClip™ Self-Ligating Appliance Prescription

Mesiodistal angulation

The SmartClip™ Self-Ligating Appliance System was designed to conform with the MBT™ Versatile+ system,[1] and follows the concept of sliding mechanics with the application of light forces and the use of a .019/.025 rectangular archwire in a .022/.028 slot.

The SmartClip™ self-ligating brackets have a rhomboidal shape and angulation is built into the bracket structure (Fig. 2.10). The system allows the clinician to perfectly position the brackets using the mesiodistal margins, incisal edges and the facial axis of the clinical crown as reference guides.

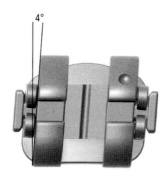

Fig. 2.10 SmartClip™ self-ligating bracket – the rhomboidal shape allows accurate positioning on the labial or buccal surface of the tooth.

Maxillary brackets

The angulation of the MBT Versatile+ Appliance system brackets for the anterior upper teeth is less than that in the original Straight-Wire™ Appliance.[3] Following the same pattern as the MBT Versatile+ Appliance System,[1] the SmartClip™ Self-Ligating Appliance provides 4° angulation for the central incisor, 8° for the lateral incisor, and 8° for the canine, thus supporting sliding mechanics and avoiding relapse of protrusion, increase in overbite, and loss of posterior anchorage.

The angulation of the upper premolar brackets is 0°, making these brackets interchangeable. This angulation also provides anchorage for the posterior teeth and intercuspation with the lower premolars, and keeps the premolars in an upright position.

The first molar buccal tube has 0° angulation, favoring a Class I molar relationship. The tube should be positioned parallel to the buccal intermarginal ridge line (see Chapter 3) to provide 5° angulation for the Class I molar relationship (Figs 2.11 & 2.12).

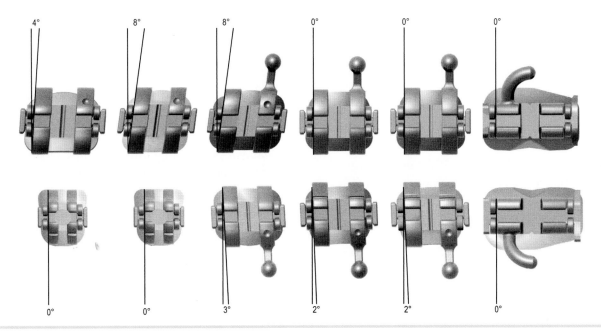

Fig. 2.11 Mesiodistal angulation of the SmartClip™ Self-Ligating Appliance upper and lower brackets (with hooks) and buccal tubes.

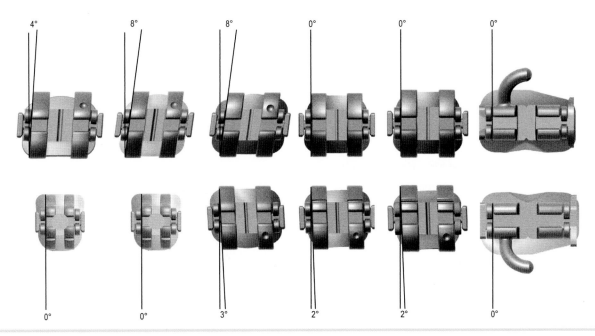

Fig. 2.12 Mesiodistal angulation of the SmartClip™ Self-Ligating Appliance upper and lower brackets (without hooks) and buccal tubes.

Mandibular brackets

The angulation of the lower incisor brackets is 0°, which helps to achieve leveling of the incisal edges and root parallelism. The 0° also angulation makes these brackets interchangeable.[1]

The lower canine brackets have a reduction of 3° angulation compared with the Straight-Wire™ Appliance values. This helps prevent protrusion of the anterior teeth and deepening of the overbite during the aligning stage of orthodontic treatment. The mesial angulation of the lower premolar brackets is 2°, which assists in intercuspation with the upper premolars.

The lower molar tubes have 0° angulation, which favors a Class I molar relationship. Tube positioning follows the same method as for the upper molars – parallel to the buccal intermarginal ridge line, providing an effective 2° angulation (Figs 2.11 & 2.12).

Inclination (torque)

During the designing of the MBT™ system,[1] changes were introduced in the torque values for the entire upper and lower dental arches. These were necessary to compensate for torque loss when applying sliding mechanics using a .019/.025 rectangular archwire in a .022/.028 bracket slot.[4]

Maxillary brackets

The SmartClip™ self-ligating bracket system features the same compensating torque as MBT™ for the upper anterior teeth, with 17° for the central incisors and 10° for the lateral incisors.[1] These torque values help sliding mechanics and allow an increase in upper arch length that helps to establish a Class I molar relationship.

For the upper canines there are two types of bracket:

● a –7° torque bracket (versatile bracket), which if rotated 180° will present +7° torque (see Chapter 3)
● a 0° torque bracket.

The upper first and second premolar brackets have –7° torque, which is the ideal value for these teeth. The left and right upper premolar brackets are interchangeable.

The upper first molar buccal tubes have –14° torque, which helps in uprighting and the control of the palatal cusps (centric cusps, see Chapter 6) (Figs 2.13 & 2.14).

Mandibular brackets

The SmartClip™ self-ligating bracket system features a –6° torque compensation for the lower incisors. The negative torque favors sliding mechanics and allows a decrease in lower arch length, thus helping the Class I molar relationship.[1]

Compared with the original Straight-Wire™ Appliance,[3] the lower canines have –6° torque (versatile bracket) (a reduction of 5°).[1] These brackets can also be positioned with 180° rotation, to give +6° torque (see Chapter 3). A 0° lower canine bracket is also available.

Lower first and second premolar brackets feature a reduction of 5° torque when compared with the Straight-Wire™ Appliance values. The first premolars have –12° torque and the second premolars –17° torque.

The lower first molar buccal tubes have –20° torque, favoring uprighting and control of the buccal cusps (Figs 2.13 & 2.14).

For the canines, brackets without hooks (versatile brackets) are also available, which can be positioned with 180° rotation.[1]

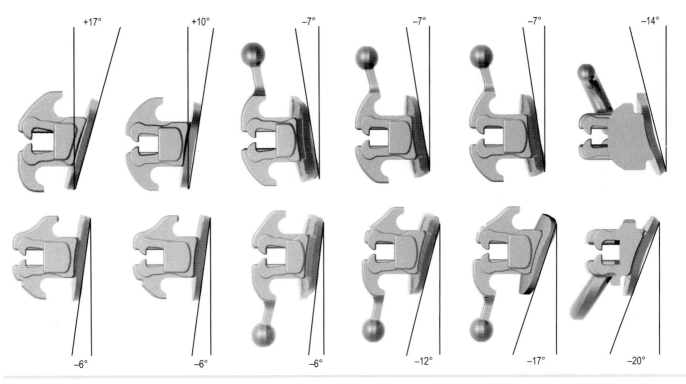

Fig. 2.13 Torque in base – SmartClip™ Self-Ligating Appliance brackets with hooks and tubes.

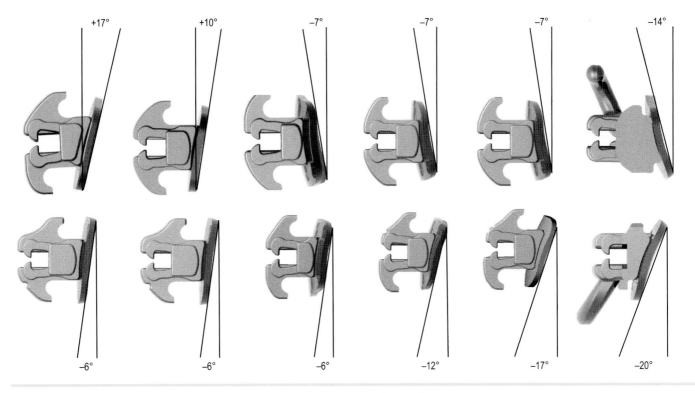

Fig. 2.14 Torque in base – SmartClip™ Self-Ligating Appliance brackets without hooks and tubes.

In–out values of maxillary and mandibular brackets

The interarch occlusal relationship in the sagittal plane is dependent on the in–out position of each tooth and the arch form used during orthodontic treatment. The in–out and the torque provide functional balance by placing the slopes of the cusps of the posterior teeth and canine marginal ridges, which are responsible for lateroprotrusive disclusion, in the correct relationship (see Chapter 6).

The SmartClip™ self-ligating bracket system does not feature rotational correction, except for the upper first molar tubes, which, as with the MBT™ system, have distal rotation of 10°.[1] Several years of experience with preadjusted appliances and the technological advances of Nitinol archwires have shown that there is no need for additional rotational control in the bracket wings.[5] Perfect contact points between teeth can be established without this (Figs 2.15 & 2.16).

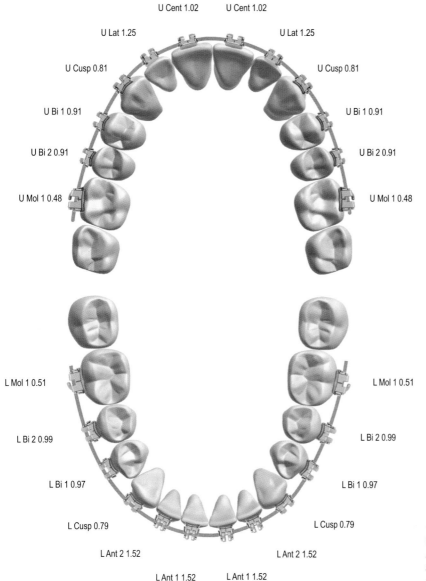

U Cent 1.02   U Cent 1.02

U Lat 1.25   U Lat 1.25

U Cusp 0.81   U Cusp 0.81

U Bi 1 0.91   U Bi 1 0.91

U Bi 2 0.91   U Bi 2 0.91

U Mol 1 0.48   U Mol 1 0.48

Fig. 2.15 Occlusal view of the SmartClip™ Self-Ligating Appliance showing in–out of brackets for the upper dental arch. The upper first molar tube has 10° distal rotation.

L Mol 1 0.51   L Mol 1 0.51

L Bi 2 0.99   L Bi 2 0.99

L Bi 1 0.97   L Bi 1 0.97

L Cusp 0.79   L Cusp 0.79

L Ant 2 1.52   L Ant 2 1.52

L Ant 1 1.52   L Ant 1 1.52

Fig. 2.16 Occlusal view of a SmartClip™ Self-Ligating Appliance showing in–out of brackets for the lower dental arch. Both brackets and buccal tubes have no built-in rotation.

Slot depth of the SmartClip™ self-ligating brackets

The SmartClip Self-Ligating Appliance is described a 'passive appliance', because the clip does not put active pressure on the archwire.[2] However, rotations should be controlled in all stages of treatment. The distance between the clips and slot surface is reduced in the lower incisor brackets compared with the rest of the SmartClip™ self-ligating brackets to improve rotational control of these teeth (Figs 2.17 & 2.18).

During leveling, use of .019/.025 rectangular archwires is recommended.

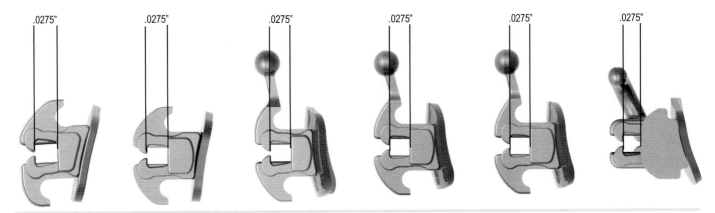

Fig. 2.17   Lateral view of the upper SmartClip™ self-ligating brackets showing the distance between the clip and slot surface.

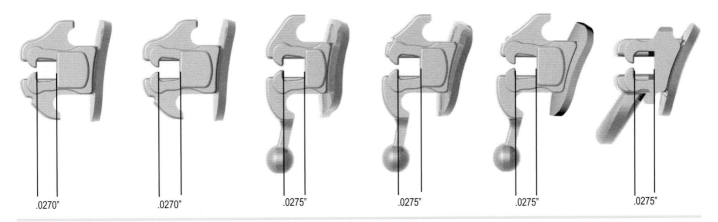

Fig. 2.18   Lateral view of the lower SmartClip™ self-ligating brackets, showing the reduced distance between the clip and the slot surface of the lower incisor brackets.

Second molar buccal tubes

Special second molar buccal tubes have been designed to be used with the SmartClip™ Self-Ligating Appliance System. The lower second molar tubes are chamfered, favoring vertical positioning and control of rotation, angulation and torque. As with the MBT™ system, upper second molar tubes are provided with 0° angulation, 10° rotation and −19° torque (Fig. 2.19) and lower second molar tubes have 0° angulation, 0° rotation and −10° torque (Fig. 2.20).[1]

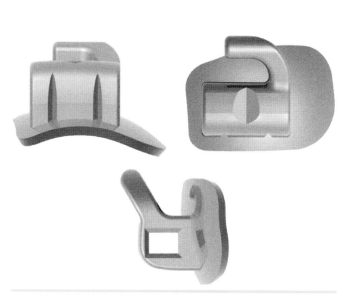

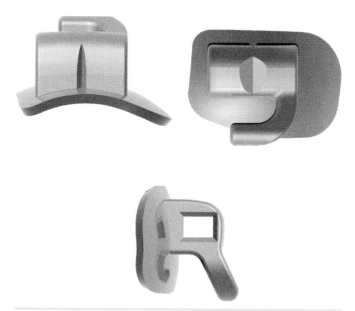

Fig. 2.19 Special tubes for the upper second molars: 0° angulation, 10° rotation and −19° torque.

Fig. 2.20 Special tubes for the lower second molars: 0° angulation, 0° rotation and −10° torque.

Special first molar buccal tubes

Special first molar upper and lower buccal tubes have been developed for use with the SmartClip™ Self-Ligating Appliance System. These tubes have a slippery surface with reduced friction that allows the archwires to slide freely in the tubes (Figs 2.21, 2.22 & 2.23).

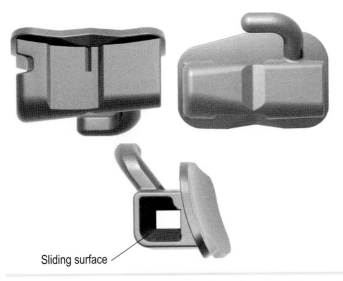

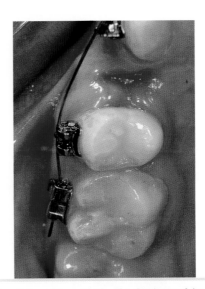

Sliding surface

Figs 2.21 & 2.22 Special tubes for the upper first molars with a slippery surface that allows free sliding of the archwire. The distal part of the tube has a groove that allows the use of metal ligatures. These tubes feature 0° angulation, 10° rotation and −14° torque. They allow easy engagement of the archwire and, subsequently, easy engagement of the archwire in the bracket slot of the second premolar.

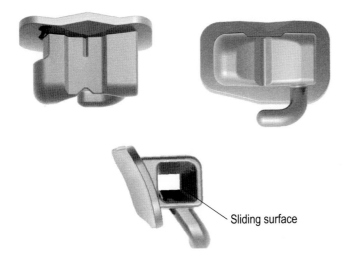

Sliding surface

Fig. 2.23 Special tubes for the lower first molars with a slippery surface that allows the archwire to slide freely. The distal part of the tube has a groove that allows the use of metal ligatures. These tubes feature 0° angulation, 0° rotation and −20° torque.

Second premolar minitubes

In first premolar extraction cases, the second premolar minitubes, developed for the MBT™ technique,[1] are ideal for use with the SmartClip™ Self-Ligating Appliance System. They are chamfered tubes and offer little friction, thus helping with sliding mechanics (Figs 2.24, 2.25 & 2.26).

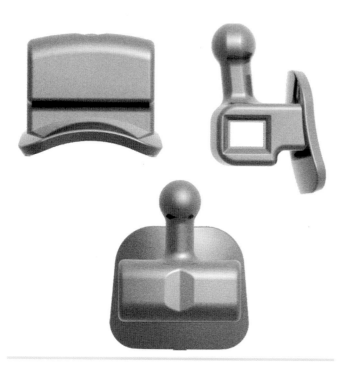

Fig. 2.24   Minitubes for the upper second premolars, allowing easy insertion of the archwire.

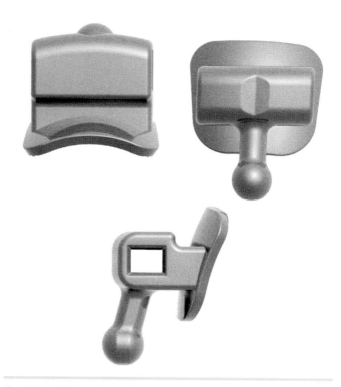

Fig. 2.25   Minitubes for the lower second premolars, allowing easy insertion of the archwire.

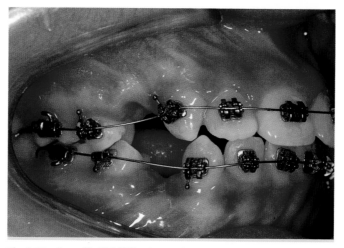

Fig. 2.26   SmartClip™ Self-Ligating Appliance: special tubes for the upper and lower first molars and a minitube on the lower second premolar.

Archwire engagement and disengagement

SmartClip™ brackets are truly self-ligating, because the clips automatically close and secure the archwire in the slot. The twin bracket design gives the clinician the option of selectively engaging the archwire with only one clip when the teeth are severely malaligned. In addition, the familiar tie-wing design allows traditional ligation if required. The SmartClip™ Appliance hand instruments have been designed to simplify the process of archwire engagement and disengagement (Figs 2.27 & 2.28).

Archwire engagement

The .014 and .016 round archwires are easy to engage in the bracket slot using either hand instruments or finger pressure. One end of the hand instrument has a rectangular notch that allows the orthodontist to direct the archwire into the bracket slot with very gentle pressure and place the wire in the slot behind the clips. When applying pressure to the wire, the clinician should support the tooth from the lingual side with his or her fingers to make it comfortable for the patient (Fig. 2.29). To make wire engagement easier, first place the archwire in the upper and lower central incisor brackets.

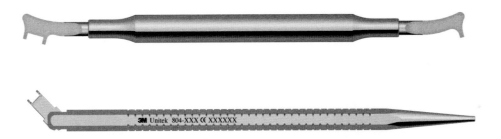

Figs 2.27 & 2.28   SmartClip™ Appliance hand instruments designed to simplify the process of archwire engagement and disengagement.

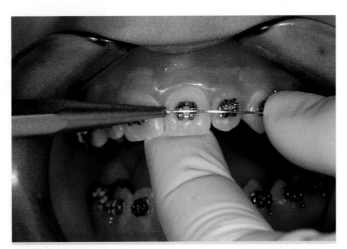

Fig. 2.29   Hand instrument for archwire engagement. When applying pressure to the wire, support the tooth from the lingual, using the finger to provide comfort to the patient.

An advantage of the SmartClip™ Self-Ligating Appliance System is that distal bends can be added to the wire before placing it into the bracket slot (Figs 2.30 & 2.31).

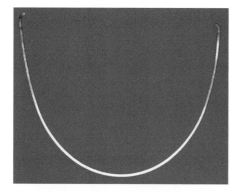

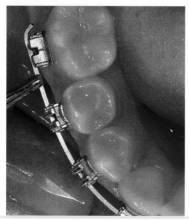

Figs 2.30 & 2.31   Rectangular archwire with bend inserted.

Figs 2.32 & 3.33   Removing a rectangular archwire from the bracket slot using the hand instrument. The hooks engage the archwire and rotation of the instrument allows leverage for removal.

Archwire disengagement

There are two hand instruments for disengagement. The other end of the instrument used to insert the wire is used to disengage the archwire from the bracket slot. The disengagement tool has two hooks that engage the wire while its central part is positioned over the labial or buccal surfaces of the mesial and distal bracket wings. By means of a rotational movement, the wire disengages from the bracket slot (Figs 2.32 & 2.33).

The other instrument is a pair of pliers specially designed for archwire removal. When the beaks of the pliers are opened, the hooks hold the archwire from the lingual with the pliers base supported on the labial or buccal surface of the bracket. When the beaks are closed, a force is generated by leverage, which removes the archwire without debonding the bracket. This procedure causes no discomfort for the patient (Figs 2.34, 2.35, 2.36, 2.37 & 2.38).

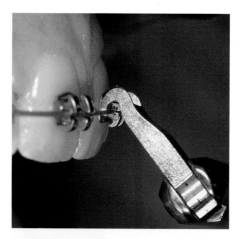

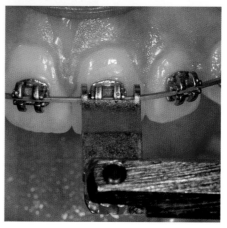

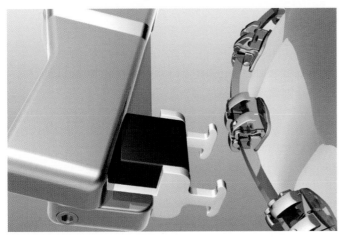

Fig. 2.34

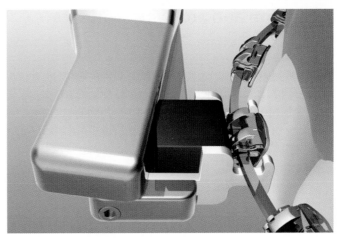

Fig. 2.35

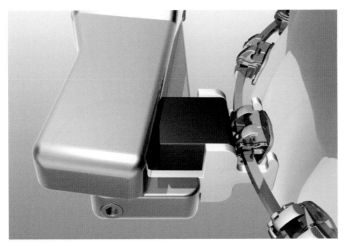

Fig. 2.36

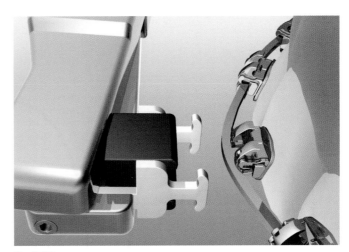

Fig. 2.37

Figs 2.34, 2.35, 2.36 & 2.37   Hand instrument designed to remove archwires from the slot of the SmartClip™ self-ligating brackets.

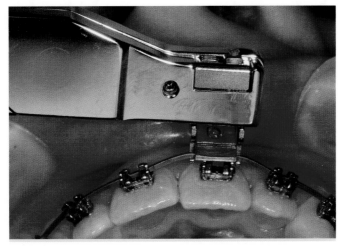

Fig 2.38   Archwire being removed with the special disengagement tool.

Arch form and archwire sequence

A major part of successful orthodontic treatment planning involves correct selection of the arch form to be used in the treatment. The patient's arch form – tapered, square or ovoid – should be checked before starting orthodontic treatment, and the final arch form should be kept close to the initial arch form (Fig. 2.39).[1]

For borderline cases (non-extraction), the expansion of the dental arches that would be possible should be carefully evaluated, because excessive expansion can lead to post-treatment instability.[6] Cephalometric analysis, the arch form, intercanine width, inter-premolar width and inter-molar width should also be considered.

The archwire sequence and the arch form used during orthodontic treatment are important for a successful outcome. Special Nitinol, stainless steel and braided archwires are available in the three arch forms – tapered, square and ovoid – for use in all stages of treatment. The archwire sequence recommended for the SmartClip™ Self-Ligating Appliance System is described in Chapter 4.

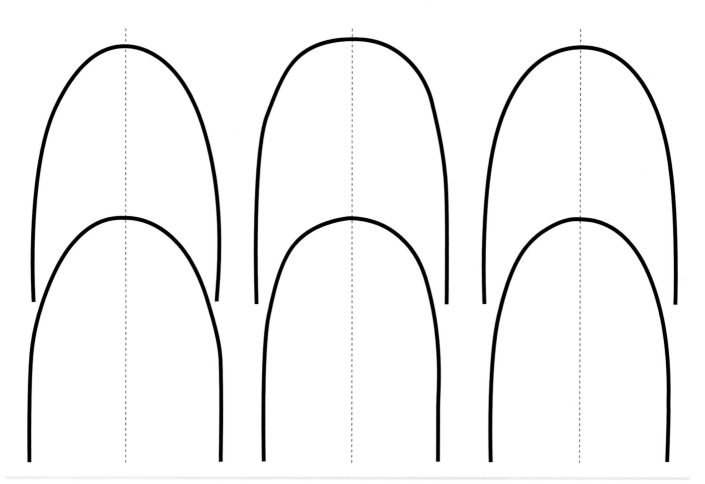

Fig. 2.39 Arch forms – tapered, square and ovoid – recommended for the SmartClip™ Self-Ligating Appliance System.

References

1. McLaughlin R P, Bennett J C, Trevisi H J 2001 Systemized orthodontic treatment mechanics. Mosby, Edinburgh, p 342

2. Trevisi H J 2005 The SmartClip™ self-ligating appliance system. Technique Guide. 3M Company

3. Andrews L F 1989 Straight-Wire: the concept and appliance. L A Wells, San Diego, p 407

4. McLaughlin R P, Bennett J C 1993 Orthodontic treatment mechanics and the preadjusted appliance. Mosby-Wolfe, London

5. McLaughlin R P, Bennett J C, Trevisi H J 1999 Bracket specifications and design for anchorage conservation, tooth fit and versatility. Revista Española de Ortodoncia 29:30–38

6. McLaughlin R P, Bennett J C 1999 Arch form consideration for stability and esthetics. Revista Española de Ortodoncia 29:46–63

CHAPTER 2 CLINICAL CASE

Name: JD
Sex: Female
Age: 11.9 years
Facial pattern: Dolichofacial
Skeletal pattern: Class I

Diagnosis

Class II malocclusion, open bite in the right premolar region, irregular incisal edges of the upper lateral incisors, and spaces between lower premolar and canines.

Treatment plan

Non-extraction orthodontic treatment using the SmartClip™ Self-Ligating Appliance with Class II elastics.

Appliance

- SmartClip™ Self-Ligating Appliance
- Upper modified Hawley wraparound retainer
- Lower 3–3 fixed retainer

Case report

The patient presented with open bite in the right premolar region, irregular edges of the upper lateral incisors and spaces between the lower premolars and canines. First, the incisal edges of the upper incisors were smoothened, and then brackets were directly bonded to the upper teeth. A .014 Nitinol round archwire was used to start aligning the teeth.

Subsequently, the lower fixed appliance was bonded and .016 Nitinol round archwires placed in both arches to finish the aligning. Leveling was carried out

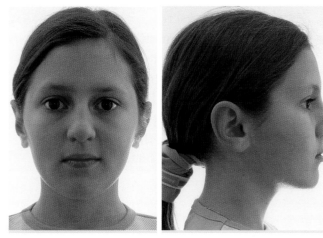

Fig. 2.40   Fig. 2.41

Figs 2.40 & 2.41
Pretreatment photographs showing Class I skeletal relationship, facial symmetry and good lip seal.

using .017/.025 classic Nitinol rectangular archwires. Space closure mechanics were used (see below) with Class II elastics and .019/.025 classic Nitinol rectangular archwires. Space closure mechanics included placing lacebacks underneath the archwires to prevent spaces from opening in the anterior segment.

Settling of the occlusion was achieved with .019/.025 braided archwires in both arches with lacebacks underneath the archwires to prevent spaces from opening up when using finishing elastics.

After removal of the fixed appliances a modified Hawley wraparound retainer was fitted in the upper arch, and a 3–3 fixed retainer was fitted in the lower arch.

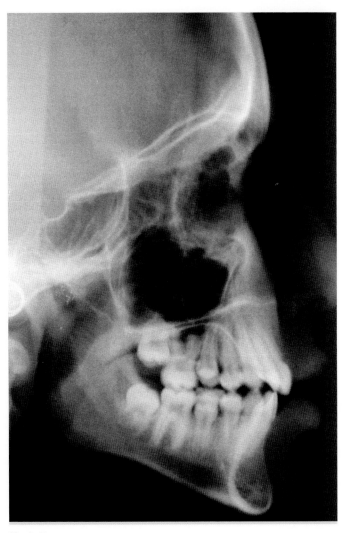

Fig. 2.42

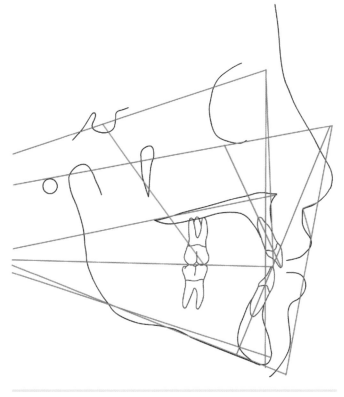

Fig. 2.43

SNA ∠	76°
SNB ∠	73°
ANB ∠	3°
A-N ⊥ FH	−5 mm
Po-N ⊥ FH	−12 mm
Wits	1 mm
GoGn SN ∠	37°
FH Md ∠	30°
Mx Md ∠	32°
U1 to A-Po	5 mm
L1 to A-Po	0.5 mm
U1 to Mx plane ∠	105°
L1 to Md plane ∠	90°

Facial analysis

Nasolabial ∠	86°
NA ⊥ nose	26 mm
Lip thickness	11 mm

Figs 2.42, 2.43 & 2.44
Cephalometric X-ray, tracing and measurements showing mild retroclination of the upper and lower incisors.

Fig. 2.44

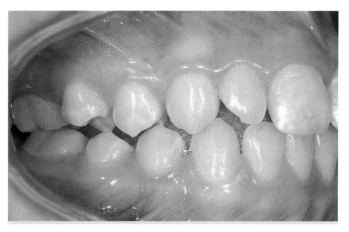

Figs 2.45, 2.46 & 2.47
Pretreatment intraoral photographs showing the Class II molar relationship, mild upper crowding, lateral open bite in the right premolar region and irregular incisal edges.

Fig. 2.45

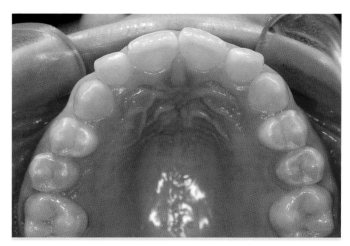

Fig. 2.48

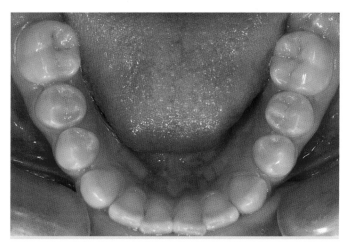

Figs 2.48 & 2.49
Pretreatment upper and lower occlusal views showing mild upper anterior crowding and spacing in the region of the lower premolars.

Fig. 2.49

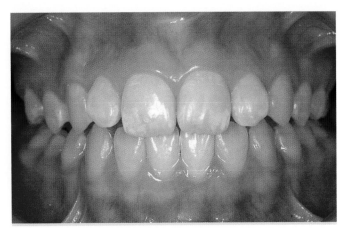

Fig. 2.46

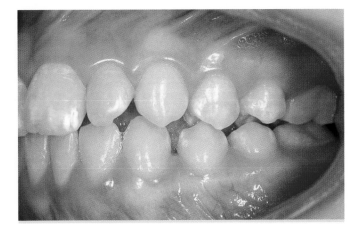

Fig. 2.47

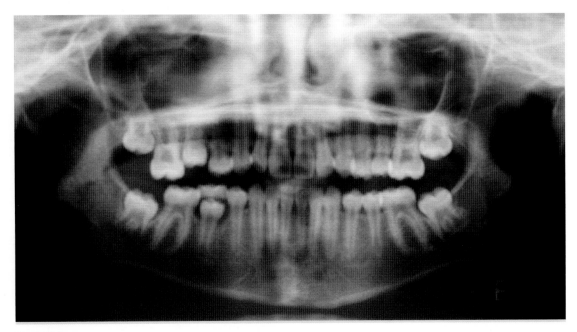

Fig. 2.50

Fig. 2.50
Panoramic X-ray showing normal eruption pattern of the teeth.

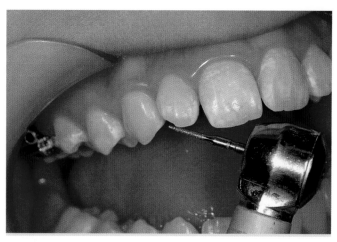

Fig. 2.51

Figs 2.51, 2.52, 2.53 & 2.54
Reshaping of the incisal edges of the upper incisors.

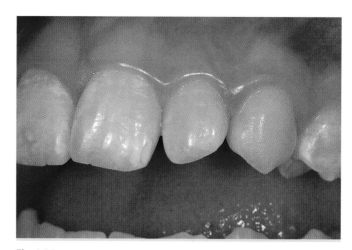

Fig. 2.54

Figs 2.55 & 2.56
Direct bonding of brackets with APC™ PLUS system.

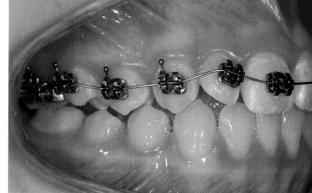

Fig. 2.57

Figs 2.57, 2.58 & 2.59
SmartClip™ Self-Ligating Appliance set-up in the upper arch with a .014 classic Nitinol round archwire at the beginning of the aligning stage.

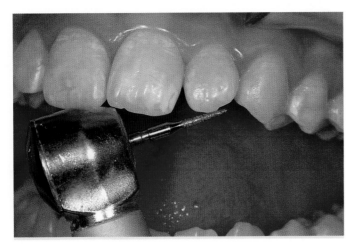

Fig. 2.52

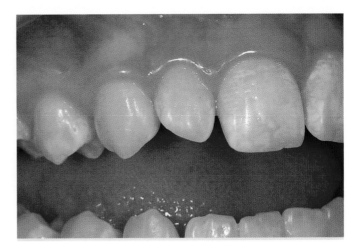

Fig. 2.53

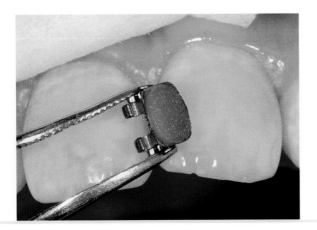

Fig. 2.55

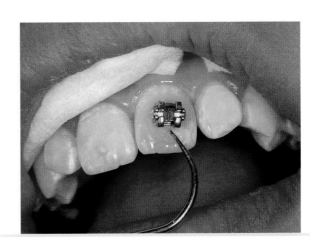

Fig. 2.56

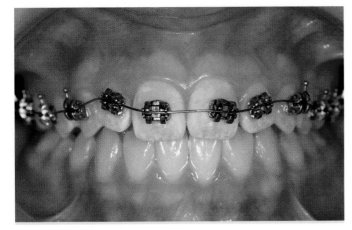

Fig. 2.58

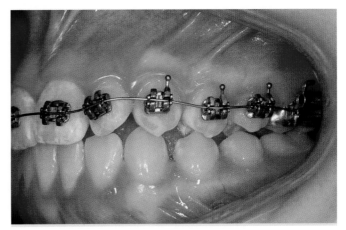

Fig. 2.59

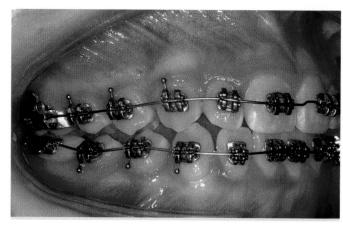

Fig. 2.60

Figs 2.60, 2.61 & 2.62
SmartClip™ Self-Ligating Appliance set-up in both
arches with .016 classic Nitinol round archwires in the
aligning stage.

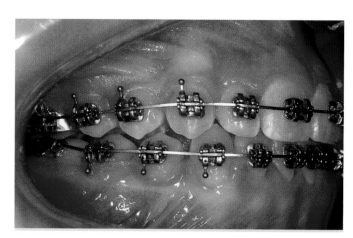

Fig. 2.63

Figs 2.63, 2.64 & 2.65
Upper and lower .017/.025 classic Nitinol archwires
for leveling.

Figs 2.66, 2.67
Upper and lower occlusal views of the .017/.025
classic Nitinol rectangular archwires.

Fig. 2.68
Heated ends of the Nitinol rectangular archwire.

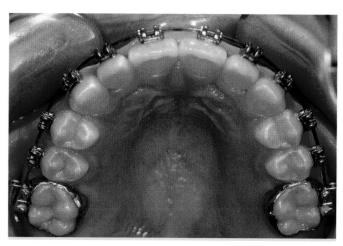

Fig. 2.66

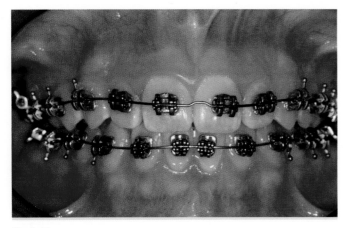

Fig. 2.61

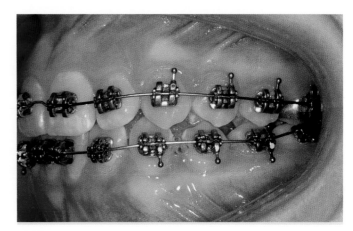

Fig. 2.62

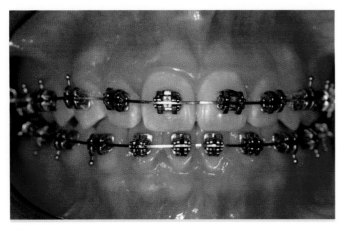

Fig. 2.64

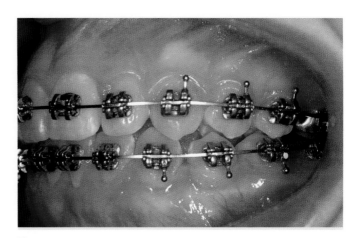

Fig. 2.65

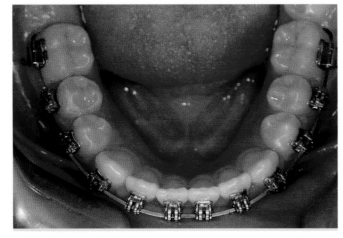

Fig. 2.67

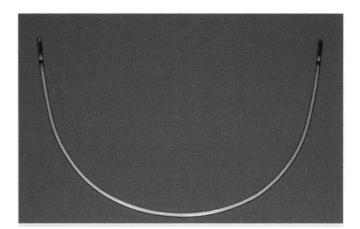

Fig. 2.68

Figs 2.69, 2.70 & 2.71
A .019/.025 classic Nitinol rectangular archwire in the upper arch with lacebacks from molar to molar. In the lower arch, the .017/.025 classic Nitinol rectangular archwire was kept in place with lacebacks from canine to canine. Note the space closure mechanics from canine to molars. Class II elastics were used on the left side to correct the midline discrepancy and the Class II molar relationship.

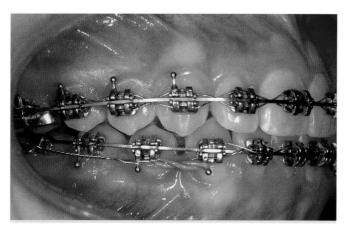

Fig. 2.69

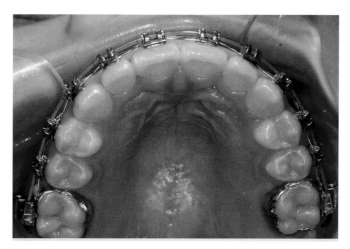

Fig. 2.72

Figs 2.72 & 2.73
Upper and lower occlusal views of the 019/.025 Nitinol rectangular archwire in the upper arch and .017/.025 Nitinol archwire in the lower arch after space closure.

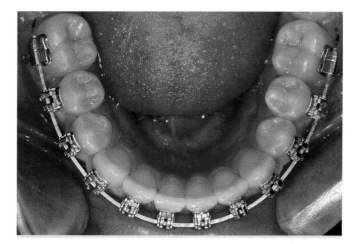

Fig. 2.73

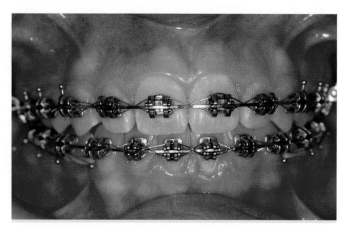

Fig. 2.70

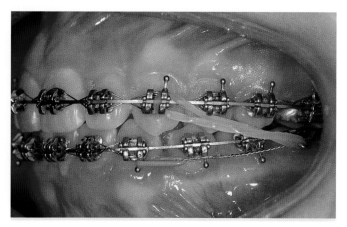

Fig. 2.71

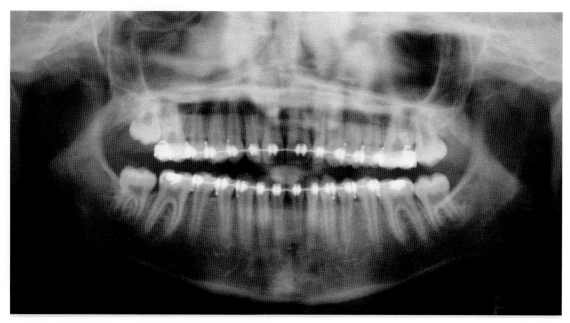

Fig. 2.74

Fig. 2.74
Interim panoramic X-ray showing root parallelism following space closure.

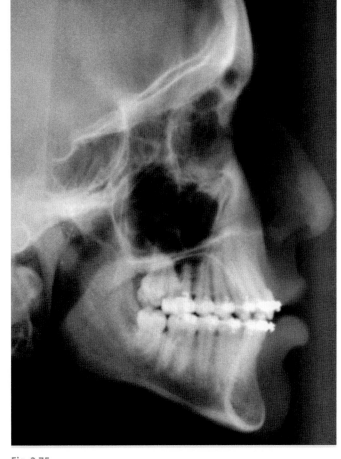

Fig. 2.75

Figs 2.75, 2.76 & 2.77

Interim cephalometric X-ray, tracing and measurements for treatment evaluation. Upper and lower incisors are well positioned.

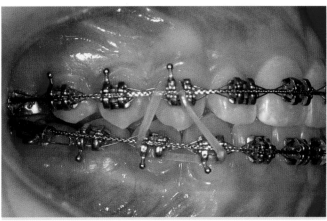

Fig. 2.78

Figs 2.78, 2.79 & 2.80
Final stage of treatment with .019/.025 braided rectangular archwire for settling of the occlusion. Metal ligatures tied underneath the archwires to prevent spaces from opening up.

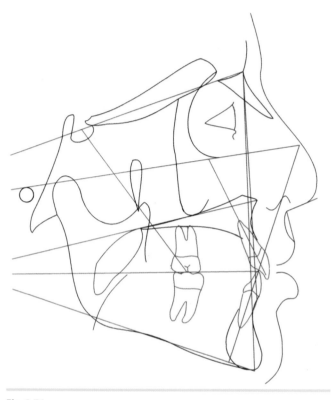

Fig. 2.76

SNA ∠	75°
SNB ∠	73°
ANB ∠	3°
A-N ⊥ FH	−4 mm
Po-N ⊥ FH	−10 mm
Wits	0.5 mm
GoGn SN ∠	37°
FH Md ∠	29°
Mx Md ∠	31°
U1 to A-Po	4 mm
L1 to A-Po	1 mm
U1 to Mx plane ∠	103°
L1 to Md plane ∠	90°
Facial analysis	
Nasolabial ∠	97°
NA ⊥ nose	27 mm
Lip thickness	12 mm

Fig. 2.77

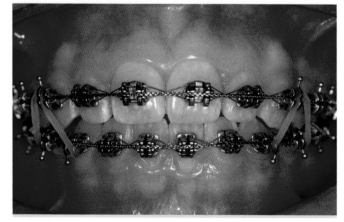

Fig. 2.79

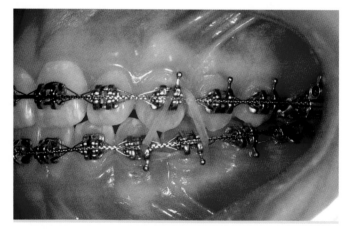

Fig. 2.80

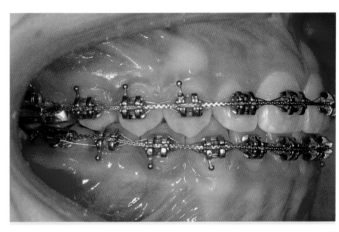

Fig. 2.81

Figs 2.81, 2.82 & 2.83
Final stage of treatment with .019/.025 braided rectangular archwire showing good intercuspation.

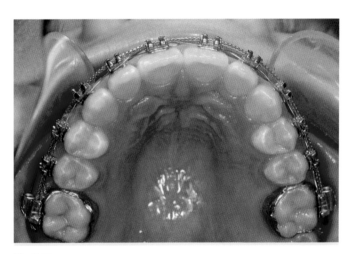

Fig. 2.84

Figs 2.84 & 2.85
Upper and lower occlusal views of .019/.025 braided rectangular archwire on the upper and lower arches. There is good alignment and arch form with well positioned molars.

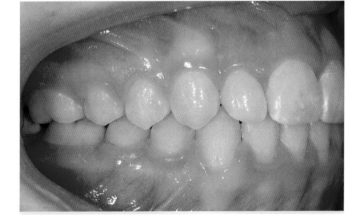

Fig. 2.86

Figs 2.86, 2.87 & 2.88
Post-treatment intraoral photographs showing Class I molar and canine relationship with the premolars in good intercuspation. The midlines are coincident with good overbite in the incisor and the canine regions.

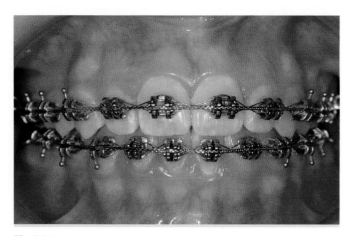

Fig. 2.82

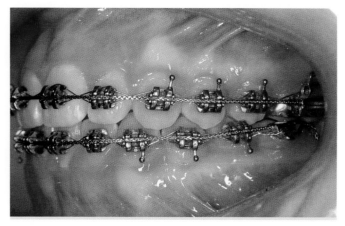

Fig. 2.83

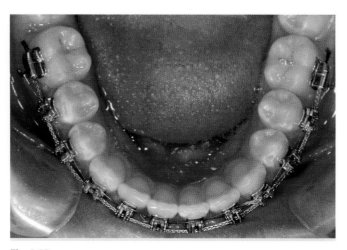

Fig. 2.85

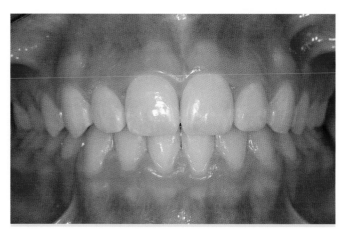

Fig. 2.87

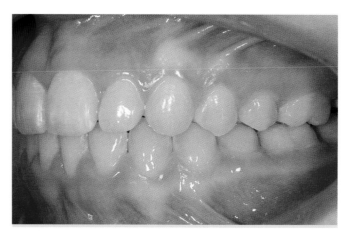

Fig. 2.88

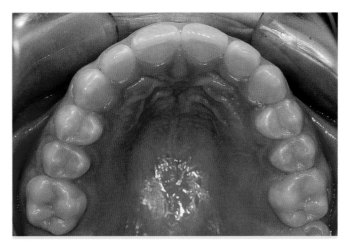

Fig. 2.89

Figs 2.89, 2.90 & 2.91
Post-treatment upper and lower occlusal views showing upper and lower arch forms and good positioning of the molars. Figure 2.91 shows the incisal guidance at the end of treatment.

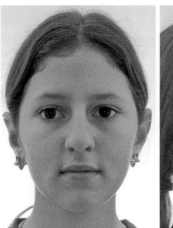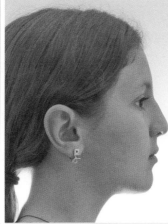

Fig. 2.92   Fig. 2.93

Figs 2.92 & 2.93
Post-treatment photographs showing facial symmetry and a good facial profile.

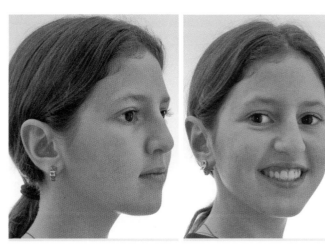

Fig. 2.94   Fig. 2.95

Figs 2.94 & 2.95
Post-treatment three-quarter view photographs showing a good smile line.

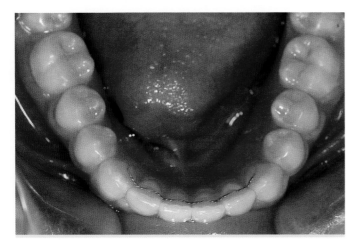

Fig. 2.90

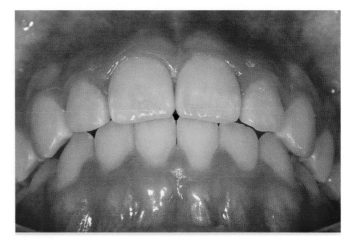

Fig. 2.91

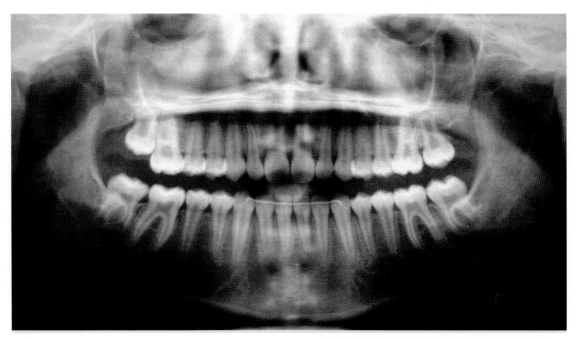

Fig. 2.96

Fig. 2.96
Post-treatment panoramic X-ray showing root parallelism.

Figs 2.97, 2.98, 2.99 & 2.100
Post-treatment cephalometric X-ray, cephalometric
tracing and cephalometric measurements showing the
well-positioned incisors. Superimposition of the initial
and final tracings shows good horizontal growth.

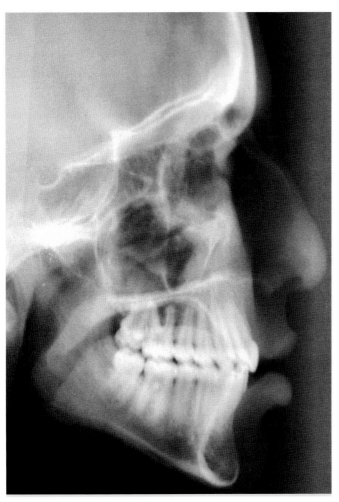

Fig. 2.97

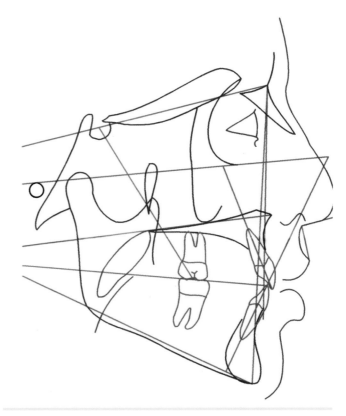

Fig. 2.98

SNA ∠	78°
SNB ∠	74°
ANB ∠	4°
A-N ⊥ FH	−5 mm
Po-N ⊥ FH	−9 mm
Wits	0.5 mm
GoGn SN ∠	37°
FH Md ∠	30°
Mx Md ∠	32°
U1 to A-Po	4 mm
L1 to A-Po	1 mm
U1 to Mx plane ∠	104°
L1 to Md plane ∠	90°

Facial analysis

Nasolabial ∠	92°
NA ⊥ nose	27 mm
Lip thickness	12 mm

Fig. 2.99

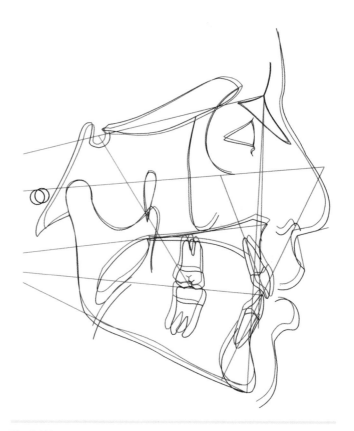

Fig. 2.100

CHAPTER 3

Customized bracket positioning system

Introduction

Since the 1970s, there has been a focus on eliminating the use of bands in orthodontic treatment. Clinicians have searched for alternative bracket systems that can speed up the setting-up of fixed appliances[1,2] and improve patient comfort.

Treatment with bands was extremely uncomfortable for the patient and also resulted in decalcification of the tooth enamel. Due to the thickness of the bands, often there were undesirable spaces in the contact areas between teeth after band removal.[3,4] However, with the evolution of composite resins and acid etching, it became possible to bond brackets directly to the crowns of the teeth. As a result, orthodontics achieved a completely new level of flexibility in the placement of orthodontic appliances, with greater precision in bracket positioning. It also increased patient comfort and facilitated the clinician's work. In addition, technologic advances resulted in improved features of the bracket base, providing superior fit and enhanced bond strength. Nowadays, orthodontic appliances can be bonded on all teeth in both dental arches, using orthodontic bonding materials. In fact, orthodontists are striving for the complete elimination of bands.

Meanwhile, one should not forget that the orthodontist's clinical evaluation is crucial for the optimal set-up of fixed appliances. Clinicians need to take into account certain aspects of each case when considering the possibility of eliminating the use of bands on molars; for example, the patient malocclusion and the need for additional anchorage. The teeth that present a higher level of difficulty during the orthodontic set-up are the second premolars and the lower first molars in patients with deep overbite, and lower molars with accentuated lingual inclination. Surgical–orthodontic cases require similar careful evaluation, because secure fixation of the appliance is necessary to avoid debonding during surgery or during the post-surgical stage.

Therefore, to achieve an accurate appliance set-up, the orthodontist should follow an appropriate protocol, checking the vertical, horizontal and axial positioning of the brackets and tubes. The bracket positioning charts[5,6] should be used as reference to avoid errors during vertical positioning of brackets, regardless of whether the direct or indirect bonding technique is used (Fig. 3.1). With the SmartClip™ Self-Ligating Appliance, either technique can be used to easily achieve a precise set-up on the buccal surfaces of the teeth.

Vertical bracket positioning

When developing the Straight-Wire™ Appliance – the first preadjusted appliance – Andrews[2] stated that the human eye is capable of locating the center of the clinical crown of a normally erupted tooth with precision. As a result, the existing devices for bracket positioning in the Edgewise technique, such as the Boone gauge, were no longer used.

Vertical bracket positioning is important in terms of the functional aspects of occlusion. To ensure accurate positioning of brackets, it is advisable to use positioning instruments (gauges) and bracket positioning charts for reference during both direct and indirect bonding techniques. Clinicians should be careful and very precise with the appliance set-up. Accuracy in vertical bracket positioning will facilitate the final stage of orthodontic treatment, because the ultimate goal is alignment of the slots of the upper brackets with the slots of the lower brackets. Overbite in the anterior region and good intercuspation of the premolars and molars are facilitated by correct vertical bracket positioning, providing good functional occlusion.

The bracket positioning technique for the SmartClip™ Self-Ligating Appliance is the same as used for the MBT™ Appliance System.[6,7] Use of **individualized bracket positioning charts** is advised for anterior and posterior teeth.

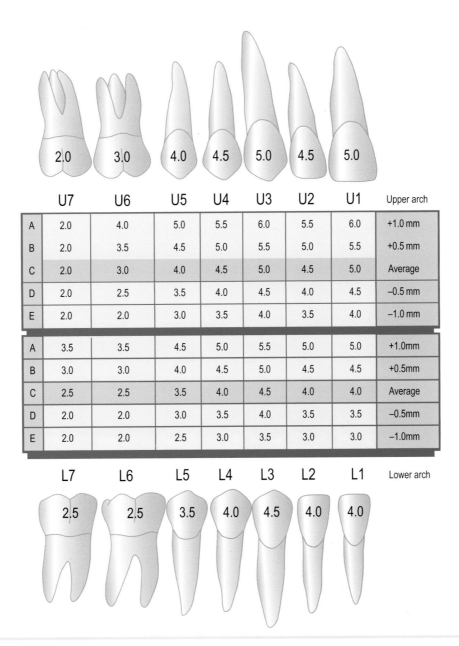

	U7	U6	U5	U4	U3	U2	U1	Upper arch
A	2.0	4.0	5.0	5.5	6.0	5.5	6.0	+1.0 mm
B	2.0	3.5	4.5	5.0	5.5	5.0	5.5	+0.5 mm
C	2.0	3.0	4.0	4.5	5.0	4.5	5.0	Average
D	2.0	2.5	3.5	4.0	4.5	4.0	4.5	–0.5 mm
E	2.0	2.0	3.0	3.5	4.0	3.5	4.0	–1.0 mm

	L7	L6	L5	L4	L3	L2	L1	Lower arch
A	3.5	3.5	4.5	5.0	5.5	5.0	5.0	+1.0mm
B	3.0	3.0	4.0	4.5	5.0	4.5	4.5	+0.5mm
C	2.5	2.5	3.5	4.0	4.5	4.0	4.0	Average
D	2.0	2.0	3.0	3.5	4.0	3.5	3.5	–0.5mm
E	2.0	2.0	2.5	3.0	3.5	3.0	3.0	–1.0mm

Fig. 3.1   Bracket positioning chart for non-extraction cases.

Vertical bracket positioning chart

In the early 1990s, to overcome the challenges faced during vertical bracket positioning when using the Straight-Wire™ technique, McLaughlin and Bennett[6,7] developed a chart for positioning brackets (Fig. 3.1). The goal was to establish a positioning system that would improve intercuspation of the posterior teeth and define the overbite for the anterior teeth. The vertical bracket positioning chart can be used as a reference for the set-up of both conventional fixed appliances and the SmartClip™ Self-Ligating Appliance.

This chapter describes a bracket positioning system for non-extraction cases, cases with extraction of the first premolars, cases with extraction of the second premolars, and atypical cases with extensive vertical discrepancy, such as open bite.

Use of the vertical bracket positioning system for the posterior teeth can lead to occlusal interferences between the upper buccal cusps and the bracket wings of the lower premolars and molars. Therefore the use of low-profile tubes for the lower molars and special tubes for the lower second premolars in deep overbite cases is recommended.[6] Such tubes allow an additional 2 mm space in the vertical plane, thus avoiding occlusal interferences during maximum intercuspation of the posterior teeth (Figs 3.2, 3.3, 3.4 & 3.5).

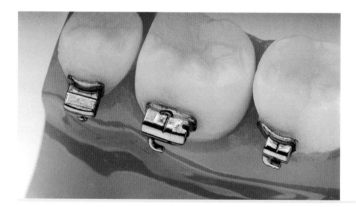
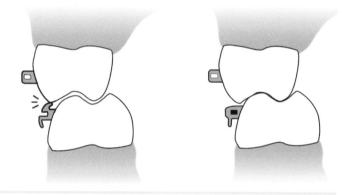

Figs 3.2 & 3.3   Special tube for the lower second premolar, low-profile tube for the lower first molar and minitube for the second molar. These accessories help to avoid occlusal interferences with the upper teeth.

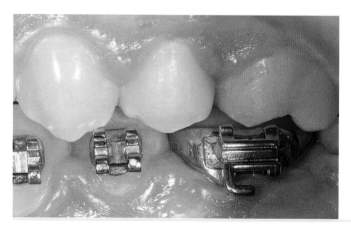
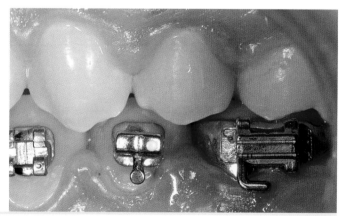

Figs 3.4 & 3.5   In comparison with a bracket, the special tube for the second premolar provides 2 mm of additional vertical space, thus eliminating occlusal interferences.

Using the bracket positioning chart

There are two systems for vertical bracket positioning.

System 1

This system, as recommended for the MBT™ philosophy, can be applied to all orthodontic cases. The clinician measures the height of the clinical crowns of all the teeth[6,7] with calipers. These measurements are then divided by two to locate, with accuracy, the center of the clinical crown. With these numbers to hand, the clinician can decide which row on the bracket positioning chart best corresponds to the crown heights of the individual patient. This row is then used as a reference for the vertical positioning of the brackets in that patient.

System 2

This system is recommended for orthodontic patients who have upper and lower incisors with normal clinical crowns.[6] The clinician should measure the height of the clinical crown of the upper central and lateral incisors and divide the values by two to locate, with accuracy, the center of the clinical crown. With these numbers to hand, the clinician can decide which row in the bracket positioning chart best corresponds to the height of the remaining teeth. The same procedure should be used for the lower teeth.

In both systems, the clinician should be aware of the possible need for some individualization due to anatomical differences in the clinical crowns of the teeth.

Recommendations for using the bracket positioning chart

Orthodontic treatment without extractions

In non-extraction cases, the average bracket positioning is recommended (Fig. 3.1).[6]

Orthodontic treatment with extraction of first premolars

When treatment involves extraction of the first premolars, the height of the brackets of the second premolars and the molar tubes will need to be varied[6] to avoid a vertical step between the canine and the second premolar. This occurs due to the absence of the first premolar, and can lead to a lack of intercuspation in this area. The height of the canines should be maintained and the brackets of the second premolars and the molar tubes should be positioned 0.5 mm more towards the gingival (Fig. 3.6).

Orthodontic treatment with extraction of second premolars

When the treatment requires extraction of the second premolars, there will be a need to vary the height of the buccal tubes on the molars[6] to avoid the occurrence of a vertical step between the first premolar and the first molar. This can occur due to the absence of the second premolar, and can lead to a lack of intercuspation in this area (Fig. 3.7).

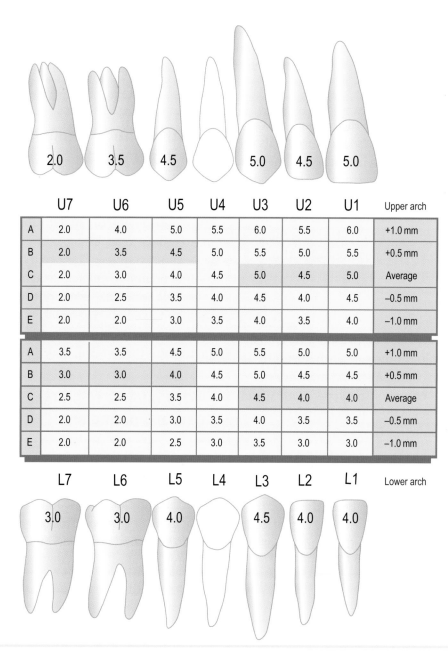

	U7	U6	U5	U4	U3	U2	U1	Upper arch
A	2.0	4.0	5.0	5.5	6.0	5.5	6.0	+1.0 mm
B	2.0	3.5	4.5	5.0	5.5	5.0	5.5	+0.5 mm
C	2.0	3.0	4.0	4.5	5.0	4.5	5.0	Average
D	2.0	2.5	3.5	4.0	4.5	4.0	4.5	−0.5 mm
E	2.0	2.0	3.0	3.5	4.0	3.5	4.0	−1.0 mm

	L7	L6	L5	L4	L3	L2	L1	Lower arch
A	3.5	3.5	4.5	5.0	5.5	5.0	5.0	+1.0 mm
B	3.0	3.0	4.0	4.5	5.0	4.5	4.5	+0.5 mm
C	2.5	2.5	3.5	4.0	4.5	4.0	4.0	Average
D	2.0	2.0	3.0	3.5	4.0	3.5	3.5	−0.5 mm
E	2.0	2.0	2.5	3.0	3.5	3.0	3.0	−1.0 mm

Fig. 3.6   Bracket positioning chart recommended for treatment with extraction of first premolars.

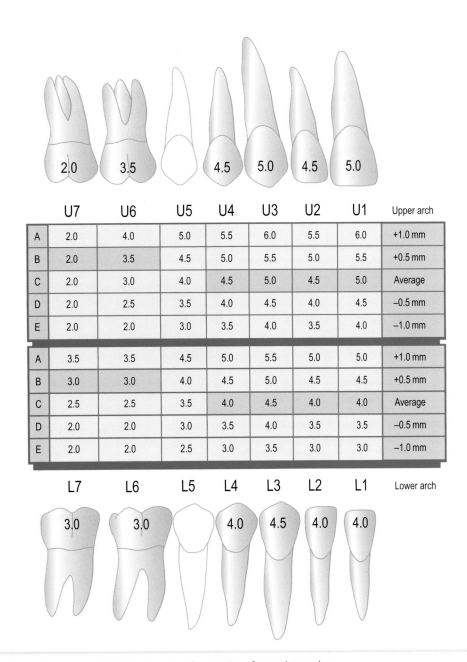

	U7	U6	U5	U4	U3	U2	U1	Upper arch
A	2.0	4.0	5.0	5.5	6.0	5.5	6.0	+1.0 mm
B	2.0	3.5	4.5	5.0	5.5	5.0	5.5	+0.5 mm
C	2.0	3.0	4.0	4.5	5.0	4.5	5.0	Average
D	2.0	2.5	3.5	4.0	4.5	4.0	4.5	−0.5 mm
E	2.0	2.0	3.0	3.5	4.0	3.5	4.0	−1.0 mm

	L7	L6	L5	L4	L3	L2	L1	Lower arch
A	3.5	3.5	4.5	5.0	5.5	5.0	5.0	+1.0 mm
B	3.0	3.0	4.0	4.5	5.0	4.5	4.5	+0.5 mm
C	2.5	2.5	3.5	4.0	4.5	4.0	4.0	Average
D	2.0	2.0	3.0	3.5	4.0	3.5	3.5	−0.5 mm
E	2.0	2.0	2.5	3.0	3.5	3.0	3.0	−1.0 mm

Fig. 3.7   Bracket positioning chart recommended for treatment with extraction of second premolars.

SMARTCLIP™ SELF-LIGATING APPLIANCE SYSTEM

Orthodontic treatment for anterior open bite

For anterior open bite cases, the height of the brackets of the anterior teeth – incisors and canines – should be changed.

The goal of orthodontic treatment is to level the planes of the slots of the upper and lower brackets, in order to obtain an adequate anterior overbite. In malocclusions with vertical discrepancies and open bites, the planes of the slots are not always level, which in turn makes it difficult to close the bite. Thus, the brackets of the upper and lower incisors and canines should be positioned more gingivally to compensate for the lack of leveling of the planes. This will help to close the bite and reduce the need for finishing elastics.

Orthodontic treatment for deep overbite

The severity of the overbite influences bracket positioning in the vertical direction. Its evaluation is important for achieving leveling of the planes of the upper and lower bracket slots (Fig. 3.8). Generally, there is no difficulty in correcting overbites, especially when the second molars have already erupted.

Individualized bracket positioning system

Upper central incisors

The clinical crowns of upper and lower central incisors show three distinct anatomical shapes[5,8] – ovoid (Fig. 3.9), square (Fig. 3.10) and triangular (Fig. 3.11). Special attention should be given to the anatomical shape of the incisors to achieve accurate bracket positioning.

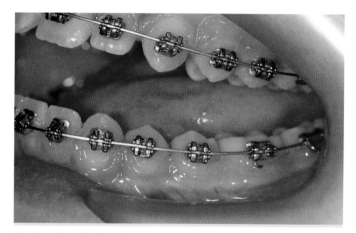

Fig. 3.8 Buccal tube positioning on the lower second molar aiming at correcting the curve of Spee and the overbite.

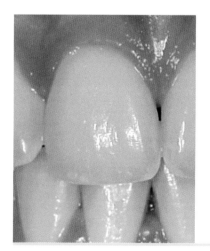 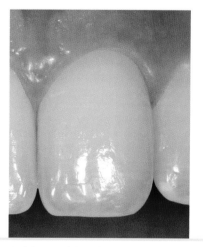 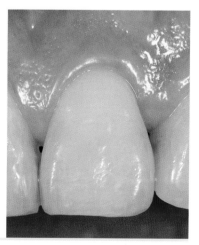

Figs 3.9, 3.10 & 3.11 The three distinct anatomical shapes of clinical crowns of upper central incisors – ovoid, square and triangular.

Andrews[2] found that the upper incisors in normal occlusions of North American individuals showed an average angulation of 3.59°. In a study by Sebata[9] on Japanese individuals, the average angulation was 4.25°, whereas Watanabe et al[10] found the average angulation in Japanese individuals was 3.11°. Trevisi Zanelato[11] found the average angulation was 2.21° in white Brazilian individuals. The average angulation based on all the research mentioned above is 3.29° (Fig. 3.12), and shows huge variations in angulation for the upper central incisors. Due to the anatomical shape and the variation in angulation of the central incisors, clinicians should pay particular attention to these teeth when setting up orthodontic appliances.

Angulation of upper central incisors in normal occlusion	
Andrews	3.59°
Sebata	4.25°
Watanabe	3.11°
Trevisi Zanelato	2.21°
Total	13.16°
Average	3.29°

Fig. 3.12   Angulation of the upper central incisors from normal occlusions as found in research conducted by Andrews, Sebata, Watanabe and Trevisi Zanelato. Also shown is the average value obtained from all these studies.

Triangular-shaped teeth require less angulation than those that are ovoid or square. The author recommends using an individualized bracket positioning system for the incisors, canines, premolars and molars.

Rhomboidal-shaped, medium-sized twin brackets with a .022/.028 slot and a .019/.025 archwire are capable of transferring the angulation built into the bracket prescription to the teeth. When positioning the bracket, the incisal edge of the tooth should be parallel to the bracket slot (Figs 3.13 & 3.14). Thus, the facial vertical long axis of the clinical crown is not the only reference used for the axial positioning of brackets on the incisor teeth. It is important to recognize that this does not apply to square and rectangular bracket designs, for example, the Straight-Wire™[1] brackets (Figs 3.15 & 3.16). In these brackets, the angulation is built in the bracket wings, and only the facial vertical long axis of the clinical crown is used as the reference for axial positioning. However, in the case of the incisors, this can result in the same angulation being imparted to all teeth, depending on the bracket prescription that has been used. Therefore, such brackets are being gradually replaced by rhomboidal brackets that provide additional reference points for axial positioning and coordinate the perspective lines into two planes along

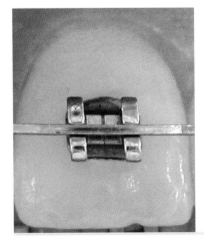
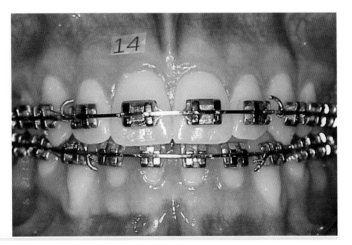

Figs 3.13 & 3.14   MBT™ brackets: rhomboidal-shaped, medium-size twin-wing brackets with .022/.028 slot and a .019/.025 rectangular archwire. Note the alignment of the bracket slot to the incisal edge of the tooth.

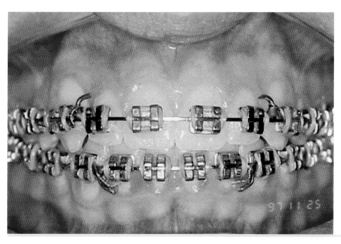

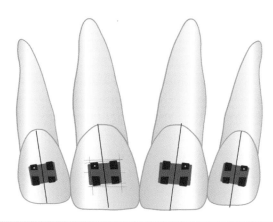

Figs 3.15 & 3.16 Rectangular-shaped Straight-Wire™ brackets with angulation built in the bracket wings: this design makes the axial positioning of brackets difficult. The lower edges of the brackets are not parallel to the incisal edges of the teeth.

with reduced bulk of each bracket.[8] The author recommends the use of rhomboidal-shaped brackets with three reference points for positioning the incisors (Figs 3.17 & 3.18).

Vertical positioning

The SmartClip™ self-ligating brackets for upper central incisors should be centered on the clinical crown when positioning the bracket in the vertical plane, as recommended for the MBT™ philosophy.[6] This positioning is very important for correcting the overbite during the final stage of orthodontic treatment to approximately 2–3 mm (Fig. 3.19).

Horizontal positioning

The labial surface of the upper central incisors is flat, allowing good horizontal positioning of the brackets. Minor mesiodistal positioning errors will not cause rotational problems for these teeth. Horizontal bracket positioning is achieved by clinical visualization, and the bracket should be centered mesiodistally on the clinical crown (Fig 3.20).[6]

Axial positioning

As mentioned above, the clinical crowns of the upper central incisors have three distinct shapes – ovoid,

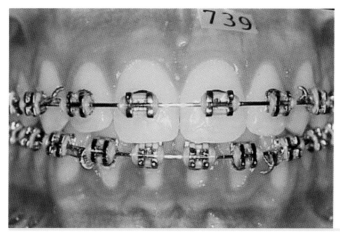

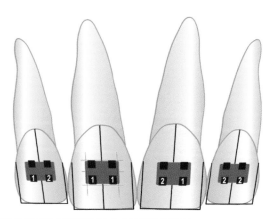

Figs 3.17 & 3.18 Full-size and medium-size rhomboidal-shape brackets, providing parallelism between the bracket slot and the incisal edges of the incisor teeth.

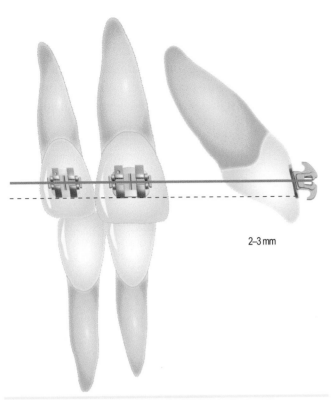

Fig. 3.19 The ideal incisal overbite is approximately 2–3 mm.

2–3 mm

square, and triangular (Figs 3.9, 3.10 & 3.11).[8] Triangular teeth should have less mesiodistal angulation than square and ovoid teeth. The SmartClip™ self-ligating bracket for the upper central incisor has 4° angulation. It can be used on ovoid, square or triangular teeth to express the required angulation for each type of tooth when applying the individualized bracket positioning system.

Axial positioning is also achieved through clinical visualization, and if the incisal edges of the teeth are parallel with the bracket slot, it indicates that the axial positioning is correct. For individualized bracket positioning for the incisors, clinicians should refer to the following: **the facial vertical long axis, the mesial and distal edges, and the incisal edge of the clinical crown of these teeth** (Figs 3.21 & 3.22). By adopting these references for the positioning of the rhomboidal-shaped brackets, a great variety of angulations considered normal for the upper central incisors are available to the clinician with a single prescription.

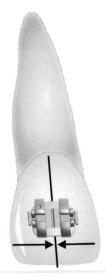

Fig. 3.20 Line to be observed for the horizontal positioning of the upper central incisor brackets – the mesiodistal center of the tooth should coincide with the center of the bracket.

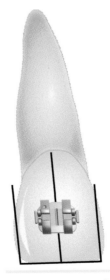

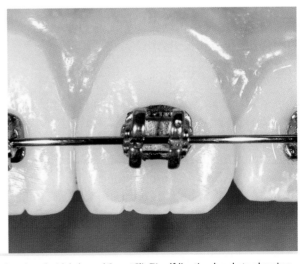

Figs 3.21 & 3.22 Medium-size, rhomboidal-shaped SmartClip™ self-ligating brackets, showing the mesial and distal wings aligned with mesial and distal margins of the tooth, and slot aligned with the incisal edge, allowing individualized bracket positioning.

However, some adjustments may be necessary if there are anatomical variations or unevenness of the incisal edges (Fig. 3.23). Such issues should be resolved before treatment, for example, by reshaping of the incisal edges to position the brackets accurately (Figs 3.24, 3.25 & 3.26).

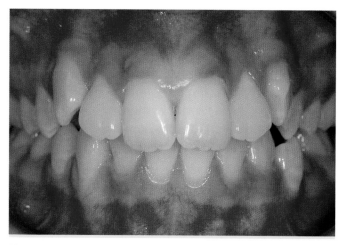

Fig. 3.23   Pretreatment photograph showing incisors with asymmetrical incisal edges.

Bracket angulation is fully expressed when a full size archwire is engaged. The bracket slot should be parallel to the upper incisal edges, which should be parallel to the lower incisal edges during protrusive functional movements (Figs 3.27 & 3.28).

Upper lateral incisors

Vertical positioning

Upper lateral incisor brackets are more difficult to position than central incisor brackets. This is due to the anatomical variations typically shown by these teeth. The size of the lateral incisors should also be considered when positioning the brackets. The MBT™ [5,6] vertical bracket positioning chart indicates that the upper lateral incisor brackets should be placed 0.5 mm more incisal than the central incisor brackets. However, in some cases, this value can be higher. The clinician should pay attention to the original

'step' between the lateral and the central incisors. During final vertical positioning of the lateral incisors, it can vary between 0.5 mm and 1.0 mm (Fig. 3.29). In cases with small or peg-shaped lateral incisor teeth, bracket height should not be compensated for during bonding. The original step should be maintained, and

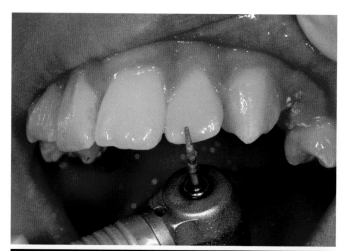

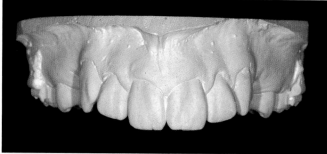

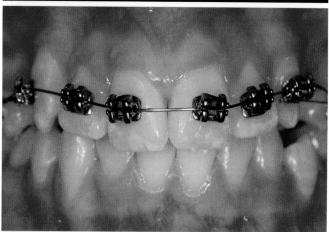

Figs 3.24, 3.25 & 3.26   Reshaping on the incisal edges for appliance set-up (indirect bonding). Cast model for indirect bonding. A .014 classic Nitinol archwire in place for aligning.

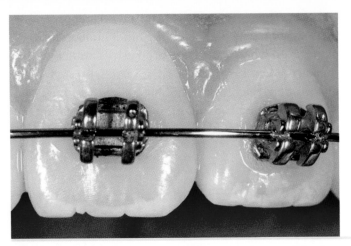

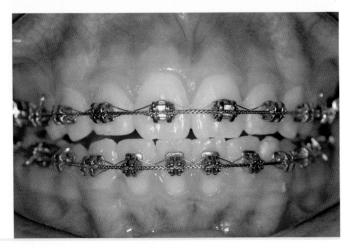

Figs 3.27 & 3.28 Final stage of the orthodontic treatment: parallelism between the bracket slots and the incisal edges. During protrusive functional movement, the upper and lower incisal edges are seen to be parallel.

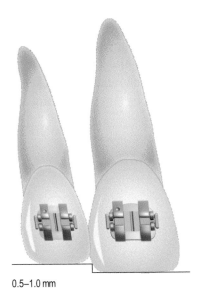

0.5–1.0 mm

Fig. 3.29 The step between the upper central incisor and the lateral incisor is approximately 0.5–1.0 mm. Bracket positioned in the center of the tooth gingivoincisally.

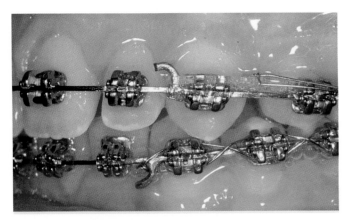

Fig. 3.30 Step between the upper central and lateral incisors of more than 1 mm.

later the crown should be anatomically built up with resin (Fig. 3.30).

Horizontal positioning

For lateral incisors with normal anatomy, the horizontal bracket positioing is guided by the mesiodistal center of the clinical crown (Fig. 3.31). Sometimes these teeth show shape variation (labial surface slightly rounded), thus making it difficult to place the bracket. In such cases, to achieve rotational overcorrection, it is helpful to position the bracket slightly toward the mesial or the distal.

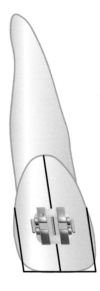

Fig. 3.31 Horizontal and axial bracket positioning: upper lateral incisor.

Axial positioning

For upper lateral incisors with normal clinical crowns, bracket positioning should be based on the facial vertical long axis and the lateral and incisal edges of the teeth (Fig. 3.31). Some teeth present shape variation, making it difficult to accurately position the bracket on the labial surface of the clinical crown. Sometimes, there is also root dilaceration, which in turn results in a root with a different angle from that of the clinical crown. This happens when, due to lack of space during canine eruption, the canine puts pressure on the lateral incisor root resulting in dilaceration in a mesial direction.

To ensure good axial positioning of the bracket, it is sometimes helpful to reshape the incisal edge of the tooth. It is also helpful to check the pretreatment panoramic X-ray before bonding the brackets for any root abnormalities (Figs 3.32, 3.33, 3.34, 3.35 & 3.36). This will allow perfect crown and root positioning, without compromising stability and

esthetics. The incisal edges of the lateral and central incisors should be parallel to the functional occlusal plane, even when there is no protrusive contact with the lower incisors (Fig. 3.28). For teeth with root dilaceration, the bracket should be slightly rotated. This will position the root in the desired angulation (Figs 3.37 & 3.38).

Upper canines

In a mutually protected occlusion at the end of orthodontic treatment, the canines should guide the lateroprotrusive functional movement. Accurate positioning of the bracket on the labial surface of the canine is therefore important to establish the correct overbite and overjet for this tooth.

The anatomical characteristics of upper canines include rounded labial surfaces in the gingivoincisal and mesiodistal directions. The reference for bracket positioning on these teeth is the facial vertical long axis of the clinical crown (Fig. 3.39).[5,6,8]

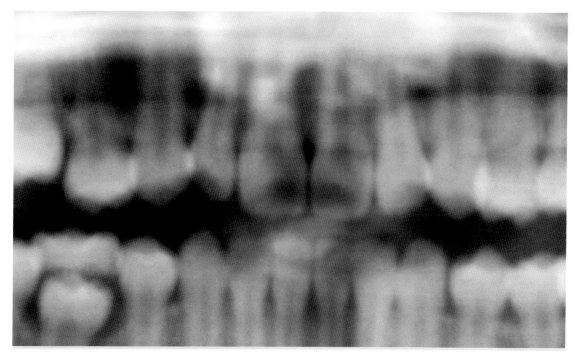

Fig. 3.32   X-ray showing the upper lateral incisor roots.

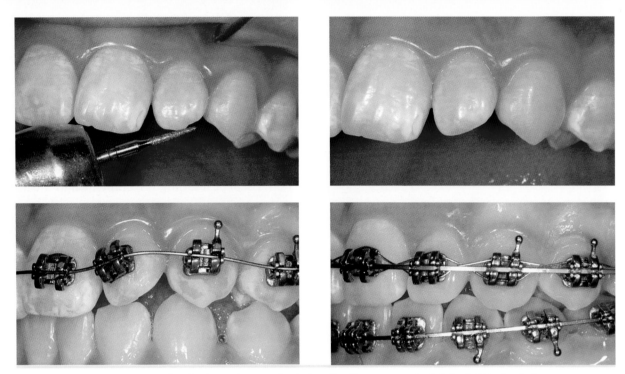

Figs 3.33, 3.34, 3.35 & 3.36   Tooth reshaping and preparation for bonding. Engagement of a .014 classic Nitinol archwire to start aligning. A .019/.025 rectangular Nitinol archwire being used during the final stage of the orthodontic treatment.

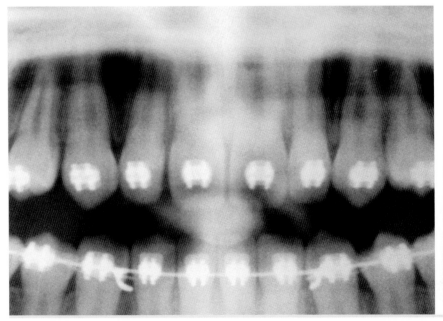

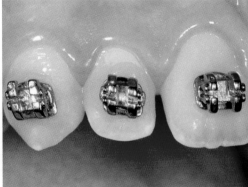

Figs 3.37 & 3.38   In cases where there may be mesial root dilaceration of the lateral incisor, axial bracket positioning can be adjusted to allow more distal positioning of the root.

Vertical positioning

It is recommended to position the bracket at either the same height as the upper central incisors (as indicated in the bracket positioning chart) or 0.5 mm more toward the gingival, using the upper central incisors as reference (Fig. 3.1). Upper canines should have adequate overbite in relation to the lower canines to allow lateroprotrusive functional movements to occur. The vertical positioning recommended in the MBT™ bracket positioning chart[5] for canines with undamaged anatomy allows disclusion of the remaining teeth on the working and non-working sides. Special consideration should be given to canines that have an accentuated cusp tip, because this could interfere with the brackets on the lower teeth during orthodontic treatment, thus compromising function and esthetics. When the canine cusp tip is very accentuated, it should be reshaped to allow better positioning of the bracket (Figs 3.40, 3.41, 3.42 & 3.43).

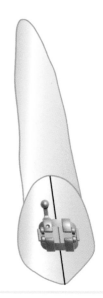

Fig. 3.39 Bracket positioning in the buccal surface of the canine, using as reference the facial vertical long axis of the clinical crown.

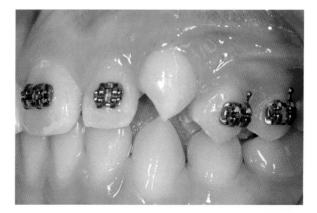
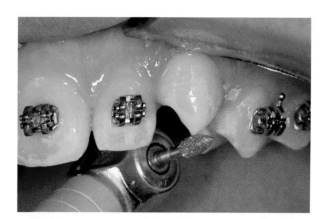
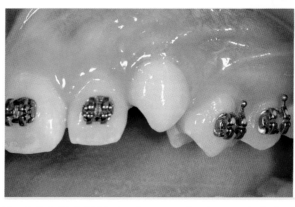
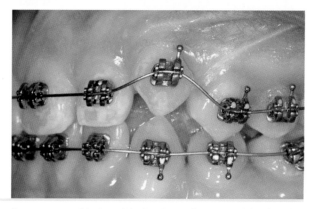

Figs 3.40, 3.41, 3.42 & 3.43 Accentuated canine cusp tip. Reshaping to allow correct positioning of the bracket in the center of the clinical crown. A .014 classic Nitinol archwire engaged to commence aligning.

Canines showing minor cusp tip wear should have the bracket positioned more gingivally to compensate for the wear, without compromising the tooth's function. For canines with major cusp tip wear, bracket positioning in the gingival direction will generate excessive tooth extrusion, increasing the labial–palatal thickness of the clinical crown occlusally, thus causing interference with the lower canine during maximum intercuspation. For these teeth, the bracket should be bonded in the usual position and the tooth built up with resin after leveling or at the end of treatment.

Horizontal positioning

Upper canines feature rounded labial surfaces, and therefore errors in bracket positioning toward the distal or mesial can result in rotation of these teeth. The center of the clinical crown should be used for horizontal positioning of the bracket[6] – the center of the bracket should coincide with the facial vertical long axis of the tooth (Fig. 3.39). Some adjustments should be carried out when there are anatomical abnormalities of the clinical crown.

Axial positioning

As the canine has a cusp tip and not an incisal edge, the anatomical reference for axial bracket positioning is the facial vertical long axis of the clinical crown (Fig. 3.39).[5,6,8]

The average angulation of upper canine crowns in normal occlusions as found by Andrews[2] was 8.4°; Sebata[9] found the average angulation was 7.7° in a Japanese sample, as did Watanabe et al.[10] In the white Brazilian population studied by Trevisi Zanelato,[11] the average angulation was 6.16°. The average angulation based on all the research mentioned above is 7.49° (Fig. 3.44). The SmartClip™ self-ligating bracket has 8° angulation, which is very close to the universal average of 7.49°, and as the twin bracket angulation is fully expressed, there is no need for additional angulation.

The 8° angulation provided by the SmartClip™ self-ligating bracket for the canines is the same as for the MBT™ brackets and allows minor rotational

Angulation of upper canines in normal occlusion	
Andrews	8.4°
Sebata	7.7°
Watanabe	7.7°
Trevisi Zanelato	6.16°
Total	29.96°
Average	7.49°

Fig. 3.44 Angulation of upper canines in normal occlusions found by Andrews, Sebata, Watanabe and Trevisi Zanelato. Also shown is the average value obtained from all these studies.

adjustments up to approximately 2° in both directions (clockwise or counterclockwise) (Figs 3.45 & 3.46). It is emphasized that bonding on all teeth, especially the canines, should be carried out using the panoramic X-ray, so positioning adjustments can be made when necessary.

Upper premolars

Due to the huge anatomical variation among premolars, special care is required when positioning premolar brackets. For these teeth, the facial vertical long axis of the clinical crown should not be the only reference used for positioning the brackets, because this could result in error during axial and horizontal positioning.

Vertical positioning

The first premolar bracket is positioned 0.5 mm more occlusally relative to the canine bracket.[6] For the second premolar, it is recommended to position the bracket 1.0 mm more occlusally than the canine, and variations in placement may be necessary due to the size of these teeth.

The buccal surface of upper premolars is generally flat occlusogingivally, and therefore vertical errors will not lead to significant changes in torque. Ideal vertical positioning allows perfect intercuspation with the lower premolars (Fig. 3.47).

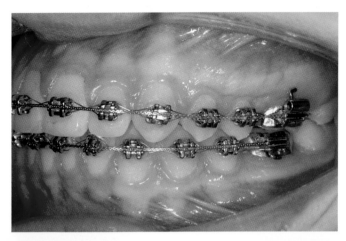

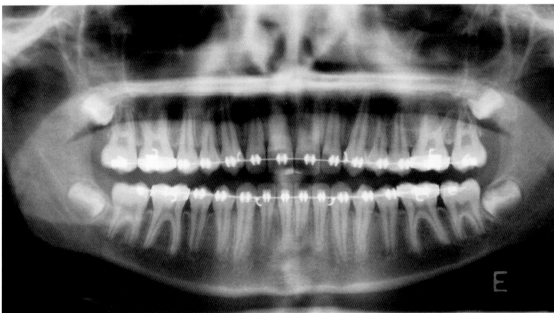

Figs 3.45 & 3.46 Final positioning of the teeth. Note the canines in good occlusion with roots well positioned.

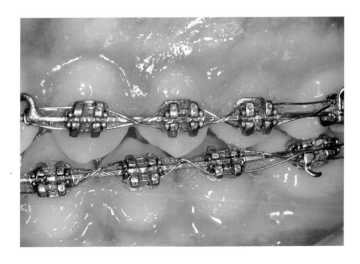

Fig. 3.47 Vertical positioning of the brackets on the upper premolars allows good intercuspation with the lower premolars.

Horizontal positioning

Correct horizontal positioning of premolar brackets is a very important part of the set-up of an orthodontic appliance. The clinician should refer to the facial vertical long axis, the buccal and palatal cusp tips, and the mesial and distal contact points. An accurately positioned bracket should help correct rotations and establish precise contact points between the premolars and the distal of the canine mesially and the mesial of the first molar distally (Fig. 3.48).

Axial positioning

The facial vertical long axis of the clinical crowns of the upper premolars does not provide a sufficient reference for axial bracket positioning and could lead to errors. Therefore, the height of the mesial and distal marginal ridges should also be used as a reference. The occlusal edge of the bracket base should be positioned parallel to a line on the buccal surface joining the mesial and distal marginal ridges – the buccal intermarginal ridge line (Figs 3.49 & 3.50).

Use of the references mentioned above for bracket positioning will avoid a step between the contact points of the premolars and the first molars. It is important to use the panoramic X-ray to check root parallelism. Due to difficulty in visualization, second premolar brackets positioning errors may occur when the direct bonding technique is used.

Upper first molars

The first molars are very important for the occlusion, therefore three-dimensional positioning of the buccal tubes should be perfect. In this way the teeth can satisfactorily perform their function as part of the masticatory apparatus.

Upper first molars should be perfectly related to the lower molars in terms of their angular, vertical and rotational positioning. The inclination of these teeth should also be taken into consideration. During maximum intercuspation, the upper first molar should show the three characteristics noted by Andrews when

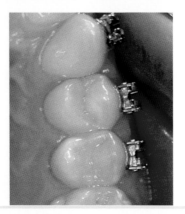

Fig. 3.48 Horizontal positioning of the brackets on the upper premolars allows good contact with the distal of the canine and the mesial of the molar.

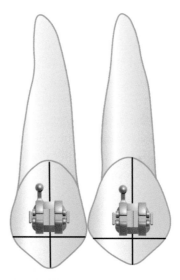

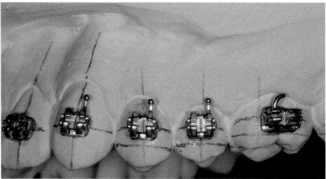

Figs 3.49 & 3.50 Axial positioning of the brackets on the premolars, using as reference the facial vertical long axis and the buccal intermarginal ridge line.

he described the first key to a good occlusion[1] (Fig. 3.51):

1. The mesiobuccal cusp of the upper first molar should occlude with the mesiobuccal groove of the lower first molar.
2. The palatal cusp of the upper first molar should occlude with the center of the mesiobuccal groove of the lower first molar.
3. The distal slope of the upper first molar distal marginal ridge should be in contact with the mesial slope of the lower second molar mesial marginal ridge.

Vertical positioning

Vertical positioning of upper first molar buccal tubes is related to the vertical positioning of the remaining teeth (Fig. 3.52). Incorrect vertical positioning of the first molar buccal tube will prevent adequate intercuspation of the premolars and canines. The center of the clinical crown is the reference for tube positioning, although it may differ if there are anatomical variations present.

Horizontal positioning

The upper first molar buccal tubes of the SmartClip™ Self-Ligating Appliance feature 10° rotation (Fig. 3.53), which is the same as for the MBT™ system brackets. Incorrect mesiodistal positioning of the tube will result in unwanted rotations. Tube positioning toward the mesial will result in additional distal rotation whereas tube positioning toward the distal will result in additional mesial rotation. The reference for positioning upper first molar tubes is the buccal groove and the center of the tube should coincide with this (Fig. 3.54).[6] Tubes prewelded to bands show this relationship, and correct mesiodistal positioning will be achieved if the band fits well on the tooth. Thus, when placing bands, the author recommends good separation of the molars to avoid problems during tube positioning.

Axial positioning

In a Class I normal occlusion, the upper first molar clinical crown is distally angulated, with the distal slope of the marginal ridge in contact with the mesial slope of the marginal ridge of the lower second molar (Figs 3.51 & 3.52). This angulation should be approximately 5° and is obtained using the 0° tube, which should be positioned parallel to the buccal intermarginal ridge line (Fig. 3.55).

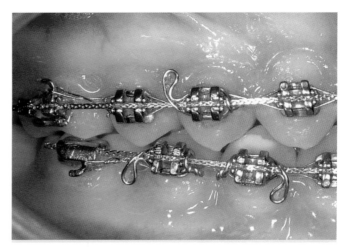

Fig. 3.51 Lateral view of normal molar occlusion showing 5° angulation and good intercuspation between the premolars and the canines.

Fig. 3.52 Ideal vertical positioning of the upper first molar buccal tubes, providing good occlusion for all teeth.

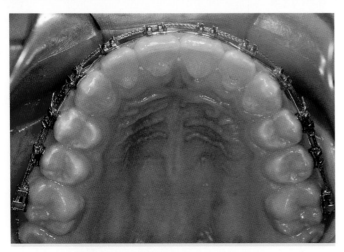

Fig. 3.53 SmartClip™ Self-Ligating Appliance: upper first molar buccal tube with 10° rotation.

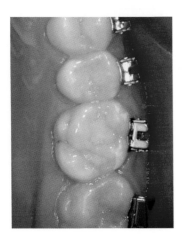

Fig. 3.54 Reference for mesiodistal and axial positioning of the upper first and second molar buccal tubes.

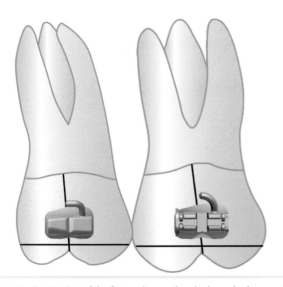

Fig. 3.55 Positioning of the first and second molar buccal tubes parallel to the buccal intermarginal ridge line.

Upper second molars

The SmartClip™ Self-Ligating Appliance System bracket prescription does not include tubes for upper second molars. Conventional tubes or minitubes are used on these teeth.

Tubes for the second molars feature the MBT™ prescription of 0° angulation, 10° rotation and –19° torque. In some cases, the angulation in these tubes will not be fully expressed, for example, due to a developing third molar in contact with the root of the second molar (Fig. 3.56). Another point to be considered is the location of the second molar in the dental arch. If the second molar is buccally or lingually displaced the force exerted by the archwire will not be enough to bring it into the line of the arch.

Thus, the critical issue with regard to the upper second molars is the expression of the –19° torque built in the buccal tube. This can be neutralized by the factors mentioned above and by inappropriate treatment mechanics that lead to buccal crown inclination (buccal rolling), so that the lingual cusps become more prominent vertically.

Vertical positioning

According to the bracket positioning chart, the upper second molar buccal tubes should be positioned 0.5–1.0 mm more occlusally than those for the upper first molars. This difference is necessary due to the smaller size of the clinical crowns of the second molars and the vertical discrepancies presented by these teeth.

For patients with open bite or a high angle growth pattern, the tubes should be positioned more occlusally, thus avoiding the possibility of extrusion, which can lead to occlusal interferences and further bite opening (Fig. 3.57).

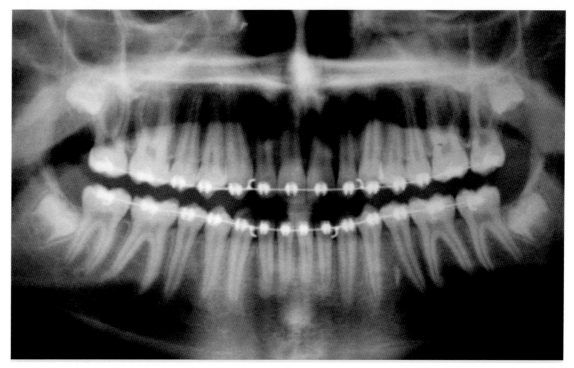

Fig. 3.56 Panoramic X-ray showing the developing upper third molars in contact with the roots of the upper second molars, making angular positioning of the latter difficult.

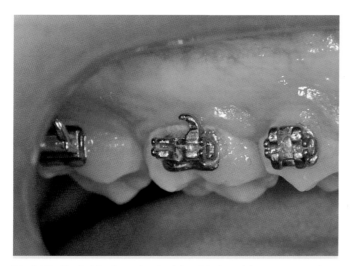

Fig. 3.57 Vertical, horizontal and axial positioning of the upper second molar buccal tube.

Horizontal positioning

The horizontal positioning recommended for upper second molar buccal tubes is the same as for the first molar buccal tubes. The center of the tube should coincide with the buccal groove (Fig. 3.58).[6] An error in mesial positioning will result in additional distal rotation; conversely, incorrect distal positioning will result in additional mesial rotation.

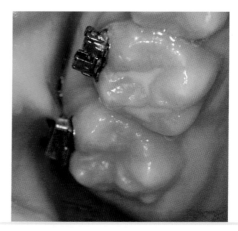

Fig. 3.58 Mesiodistal positioning of the upper second molar buccal tube.

Axial positioning

Axial positioning of the upper second molar buccal tubes follows the same protocol recommended for the upper first molar buccal tubes. The tube should be placed parallel to the buccal intermarginal ridge line to provide 5° distal angulation.[6,12] This 5° angulation is often compromised by the third molar if it is in contact with the root of the second molar (Fig. 3.55). However, the second molar can be ideally positioned after the extraction of the third molar, or when enough space is available for the eruption of the third molar.

Lower central and lateral incisors

The clinical crowns of the lower incisors, as those of the upper incisors mentioned earlier in this chapter, have three distinct shapes – ovoid, square, and triangular.[8] When evaluating the functional aspects of a normal occlusion at the end of orthodontic treatment, the incisal edges of the lower incisors should be parallel to the functional occlusal plane and to the incisal edges of the upper incisors (Fig. 3.28).

Andrews[2] found that the lower central incisors in normal occlusions showed an average angulation of 0.56° and showed the lateral incisors 0.38°. Sebata[9] found the average angulation of the lower central incisors was –0.48° and of the lateral incisors was –1.20° whereas Watanabe et al[10] reported values of 2.0° and 2.3°, respectively. Trevisi Zanelato[11] found the average angulation was 0.03° for the central incisor and –0.58° for the lateral incisor. The average angulation based on the research mentioned above is 0.51° for the central incisors and –0.23° for the lateral incisors (Fig. 3.59).

Vertical positioning

For all four lower incisors, the bracket should be positioned vertically at the center of the clinical crown (Fig. 3.60). Alignment of these teeth is very sensitive to vertical positioning, and even minor positioning errors will lead to steps between the teeth. In teeth with abnormalities of the incisal edge, these should be reshaped before placing the brackets. The labial surfaces of these teeth are generally flat in the vertical direction, allowing a good fit of the bracket base to the tooth, without interfering with the torque. The overbite can often compromise the positioning of the brackets on these teeth. In such cases, the author recommends correcting the overbite first by starting the treatment in the upper arch and, after correction of the overbite, proceeding with bonding the lower arch.

In anterior open bite cases, the lower incisor brackets should be positioned more gingivally.[6]

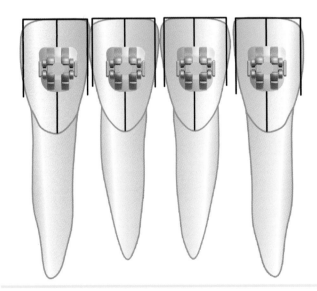

Angulation of lower central and lateral incisors in normal occlusion		
	Central	Lateral
Andrews	0.56°	0.58°
Sebata	–0.48°	–1.20°
Watanabe	2.00°	2.30°
Trevisi Zanelato	–0.03°	–0.58°
Total	2.05°	1.10°
Average	0.51°	0.28°

Fig. 3.59 Angulation values of the lower incisors in normal occlusions as found in research conducted by Andrews, Sebata, Watanabe and Trevisi Zanelato. Also shown is the average value obtained from all these studies.

Fig. 3.60 For the lower incisors, the bracket should be centered on the buccal surface of the clinical crown both horizontally and vertically, that is, in the gingivo-incisal and mesiodistal directions.

Horizontal positioning

Precise horizontal positioning of lower incisor brackets is important due to the risk of rotations. The buccal surface of the incisor teeth has a rounded shape in the mesiodistal direction, and bracket positioning toward the distal or mesial will result in rotation of these teeth.

The mesial and distal wings of the SmartClip™ self-ligating bracket should be centered on the labial surface of the clinical crown in the mesiodistal direction (Fig. 3.60). The lateral incisors require special attention due to the possibility of anatomical variations that can lead to rotational errors.

Axial positioning

Twin brackets perform well in achieving the final axial positions of the lower incisors (Figs 3.61 & 3.62). Brackets with 0° angulation are recommended to obtain root parallelism of the lower incisors (Fig. 3.63).[6] To achieve this, the facial vertical long axis, the incisal edges, and the lateral surfaces of the clinical crowns of the incisors need to be taken into account (Fig. 3.60). The panoramic X-ray is indispensable during bonding, especially for lateral incisors whose roots can vary in shape due to lack of space during eruption.

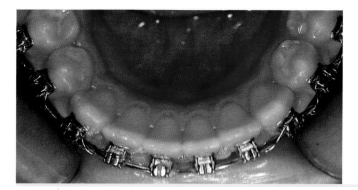 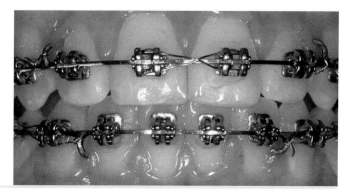

Figs 3.61 & 3.62   Horizontal and axial positioning of brackets on the lower incisor teeth.

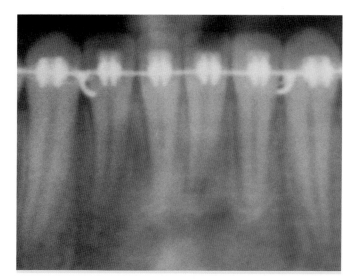

Fig. 3.63   End of treatment radiograph showing the alignment of the roots of the lower incisors bonded with 0° brackets.

Lower canines

Upper and lower canines are very important teeth for functional occlusion, because they allow mutually protected occlusion during lateroprotrusive movements. For the lower canines, −6° torque allows centering the roots in the mandibular alveolar bone, which results in better occlusion between the upper and lower canines during lateroprotrusive movements.[6]

Vertical positioning

Lower canines have a rounded labial surface in the gingivoincisal direction and bracket positioning errors in this direction result in incorrect torque. For teeth with normal anatomy, the bracket should be positioned at the center of the clinical crown (Fig. 3.64). In the vertical plane, lower canine brackets should be positioned approximately 0.5 mm more gingivally than the incisors (Fig. 3.1).[6]

In cases of canines with worn cusp tips, the clinician should consider either reshaping the enamel or positioning the bracket a little further toward the gingival. It is important to recognize that positioning the bracket more gingivally will result in an increase in negative torque, tipping the clinical crown lingually.

Horizontal positioning

Lower canines have a rounded labial surface in the mesiodistal direction. To achieve the recommended mesiodistal position, the lower canine bracket should be centered on the buccal surface of the tooth, using the facial vertical long axis, to allow the contact point of the canine to make correct contact with the distal contact point of the lateral incisor and with the mesial contact point of the premolars (Figs 3.65 & 3.66).

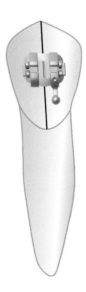

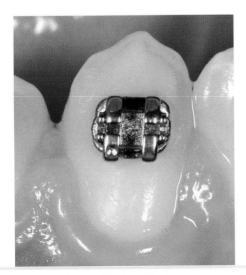

Fig. 3.64 Correct vertical positioning of the lower canine bracket.

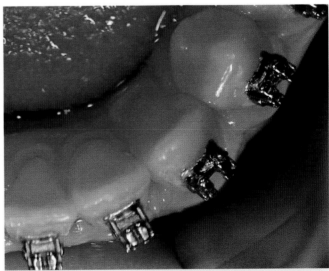

Figs 3.65 & 3.66 Horizontal and axial positioning of the lower canine bracket. Note the alignment with the facial vertical long axis of the clinical crown.

Axial positioning

The anatomical reference for axial positioning of lower canine brackets is the facial vertical long axis of the clinical crown. The mesial and distal wings should be parallel to the facial vertical long axis of the clinical crown (Fig. 3.65).[6]

Andrews[2] found that the average angulation for lower canines in normal occlusions was 2.48°. Sebata[9] found the average angulation in a Japanese sample was 1.48°, whereas in the study by Watanabe et al[10] it was 5.4°. For the white Brazilian population, Trevisi Zanelato[11] found the average angulation was 2.43°. The overall average angulation based on the research mentioned above is 2.95° (Fig. 3.67).

The SmartClip™ Self-Ligating Appliance lower canine brackets have 3° angulation for achieving correct axial positioning of the tooth. The brackets allow adjustments from +2° to –2° in the axial direction. A panoramic X-ray is helpful when positioning lower canine brackets to check for minor axial adjustments that may be required.

Lower premolars

Lower premolars require extra care during bracket positioning. It is not sufficient to rely on the facial vertical long axis. Anatomical characteristics of the premolars need be considered to achieve good three-dimensional positioning of the teeth.

Vertical positioning

The buccal surface of the clinical crown of the lower premolars is rounded in the occlusogingival direction. Errors in the vertical direction effectively change the torque built in the bracket. The recommended vertical positioning for the first premolars is the same as that for the lower incisors. For the second premolar it is correct to position the bracket 0.5 mm more toward the occlusal.[6] Correct vertical positioning of these teeth leads to better intercuspation with the upper premolars (Fig. 3.68).

Horizontal positioning

The buccal surface of the lower premolars is rounded in the mesiodistal direction, and accurate mesiodistal bracket positioning helps to avoid rotation of these teeth. In most cases, the facial vertical long axis of the clinical crown is not enough as a reference for good bracket positioning. The mesial and distal contact points of the tooth and the two buccal and lingual cusp tips should also be considered. Horizontal bracket positioning should establish adequate contact points between the premolars, as well as with the distal of the canine and the mesial of the first molar (Figs 3.69 & 3.70).

Angulation of lower canines in normal occlusion	
Andrews	2.48°
Sebata	1.48°
Watanabe	5.40°
Trevisi Zanelato	2.43°
Total	11.79°
Average	2.95°

Fig. 3.67 Angulation values of the upper central incisors in normal occlusions as found by Andrews, Sebata, Watanabe and Trevisi Zanelato. Also shown is the average value obtained from all these studies.

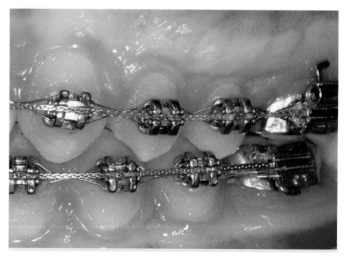

Fig. 3.68 Vertical positioning of lower premolar brackets providing good posterior intercuspation at the end of the orthodontic treatment.

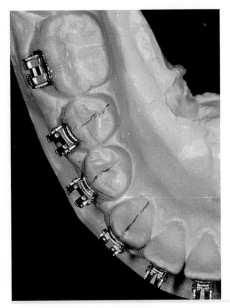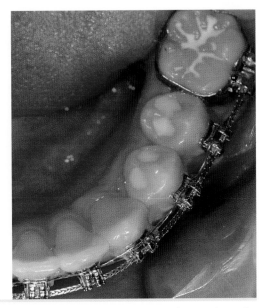

Figs 3.69 & 3.70 Horizontal positioning on the lower premolars: the facial vertical long axis, the cusp tips and the points of contact are used for reference.

Axial positioning

Axial bracket positioning for premolars is difficult to accomplish because of the difficulty in visualizing these teeth during direct bonding.

For correct bracket positioning of premolars, the clinician should focus on the facial vertical long axis and the mesial and distal marginal ridges. A line connecting the two ridges (buccal intermarginal ridge line) should be traced on the buccal surface, and this should be parallel to the occlusal edge of the bracket base (Fig. 3.71). This allows perfect contact between the premolars, and with the distal of the canines, and the mesial of the first molars. The panoramic X-ray should be checked to ensure root parallelism during bracket positioning.

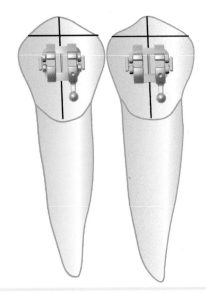

Fig. 3.71 Axial positioning on the lower premolars: the facial vertical long axis and the buccal intermarginal ridge line are used for reference.

Lower first molars

Inadequate positioning of the lower first molars can occur due to failure to achieve correct horizontal positioning of the buccal tubes of the preadjusted appliance.

Vertical positioning

Vertical bracket positioning of first molars is often compromised by the overbite or by the severe lingual inclination of these teeth in cases with a steep curve of Wilson.[13] Inaccurate tube positioning in the gingival direction can result in negative torque, altering the first molar relationship with the premolar. The occlusal wings of the tubes should be ground down to allow ideal placement in the occlusogingival direction in such cases.

The SmartClip™ Self-Ligating Appliance System features low-profile tubes for lower first molars, which help in achieving ideal vertical positioning[14] (Fig. 3.72).

Horizontal positioning

First molars can get badly rotated as a result of inaccurate horizontal positioning of the tube.

Lower first molars should have 0° rotation, which provides good mesial and distal contact points and helps establish good occlusion with the upper first molars. Often the mesial cusp is not the correct reference for horizontal positioning of the tube to maintain the molars in 0° rotation. In larger teeth, the first molars have a central buccal cusp which is very prominent buccally; consequently, if the mesial cusp is used as the reference for positioning the tube, there will be lingual rotation (Fig. 3.73). To avoid the occurrence of this type of rotation, the tube should be positioned in the center of the buccal surface of the tooth (Fig. 3.74).

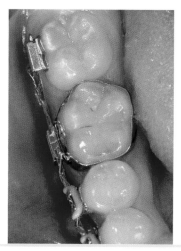

Fig. 3.73 Error in the horizontal positioning of the buccal tube in the mesial direction leading to molar rotation.

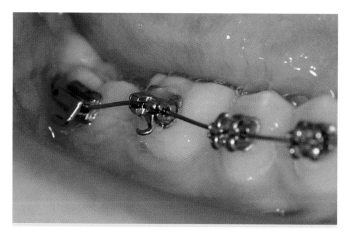

Fig. 3.72 Positioning of a low-profile buccal tube on the lower first molar, providing 2 mm of additional vertical space.

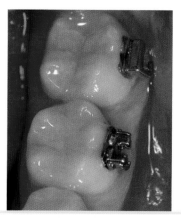

Fig. 3.74 Recommended positioning for buccal tubes: the center of the buccal surface of the lower first molar and second molar is used as a reference leading to 0° rotation.

With regard to bands, the buccal tube should be welded toward the distal, so that the opening of the tube and the lingual margin of the band are parallel, depending on the tooth's anatomy (Figs 3.75 & 3.76).

Axial positioning

Lower molars should show 2° mesial inclination and this is achieved by positioning the buccal tube parallel with the buccal intermarginal ridge line (Figs 3.77 & 3.78).[6]

When using conventional tubes welded to bands, they should be welded parallel to the occlusal edge of the bands. In the mouth, the bands should then be placed parallel to the buccal intermarginal ridge line (Fig. 3.79).

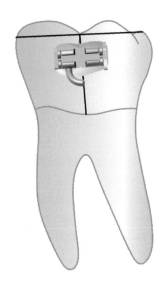

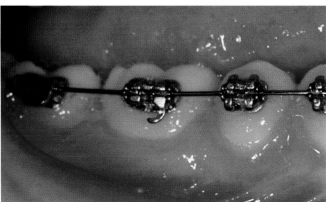

Figs 3.77 & 3.78   Axial positioning of the lower first molar buccal tube. It should be placed parallel to the buccal intermarginal ridge line, providing 2° angulation.

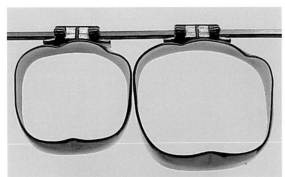

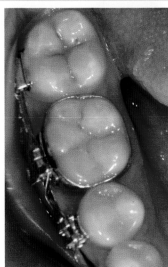

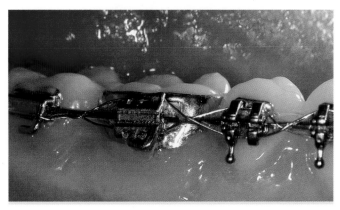

Figs 3.75 & 3.76   Buccal tube welded to the band, establishing 0° rotation for the lower first molar.

Fig. 3.79   It is recommended placing the bands parallel to the buccal intermarginal ridge line.

Lower second molars

Lower second molars are important teeth in orthodontic biomechanics and the final stage of orthodontic treatment. They normally have a well defined anatomical shape with two buccal cusps, which facilitates the positioning of the buccal tubes. The positioning challenge lies in the difficult access to the buccal surface of these teeth during direct bonding. Minitubes, developed especially for the MBT™ technique, allow positioning in relation to the mesial cusp. This in turn allows early inclusion of the lower second molars in the orthodontic treatment (Fig. 3.80).

Vertical positioning

The lower second molar buccal tube should be centered vertically on the clinical crown (Fig. 3.1). Incorrect vertical positioning will result in a step between the second molar and the first molar, resulting in occlusal interferences during functional movements. Low-profile tubes or minitubes are a good option in cases with deep overbite or severe inclination of the curve of Wilson.[13]

Horizontal positioning

Lower second molar buccal tubes have 0° rotation, which allows good contact with the lower first molars and good occlusion with the upper second molars.

Lower second molars have two buccal cusps, and these are used to locate the tube position in the mesiodistal direction. It is recommended that the center of the tube should coincide with the buccal groove of the clinical crown to avoid unwanted rotations (Fig. 3.74).[6]

Axial positioning

Tubes for lower second molars have 2° angulation and the axial positioning protocol is similar to that used for the buccal tubes of the first molars.[6] The bands and/or buccal tubes should be placed parallel to the buccal intermarginal ridge line (Fig. 3.81).

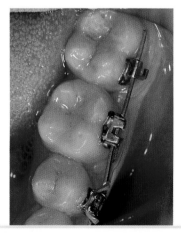

Fig. 3.80 Minitube (MBT™ prescription) positioned using as reference the mesial cusp of the lower second molar.

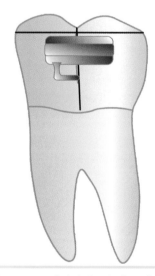

Fig. 3.81 It is recommended placing the buccal tube parallel to the buccal intermarginal ridge line in order to obtain 2° angulation for the lower second molar.

References

1. Andrews L F 1976 The Straight-Wire appliance origin, controversy, commentary. Journal of Clinical Orthodontics 10:99–114

2. Andrews L F 1989 Straight-Wire: the concept and appliance. L A Wells, San Diego, p 407

3. Angle E H 1928 The latest and best in orthodontic mechanism. Dental Cosmos 70:1143–1158

4. Angle E H 1929 The latest and best in orthodontic mechanism. Dental Cosmos 71:260–270

5. Bennett J C, McLaughlin R P 1999 Practical techniques for achieving improved accuracy in bracket positioning. Revista Española de Ortodoncia 29:39–45

6. McLaughlin R P, Bennett J C, Trevisi H J 2001 Systemized orthodontic treatment mechanics. Mosby, Edinburgh

7. McLaughlin R P, Bennett J C, Trevisi H J 1999 Bracket specifications and design for anchorage conservation, tooth fit and versatility. Revista Española de Ortodoncia 29:30–8

8. McLaughlin R P, Bennett J C 1997 Orthodontic treatment mechanics and the preadjusted appliance. Isis Medical Media, Oxford. Republished in 2002 by Mosby, Edinburgh

9. Sebata E 1980 An orthodontic study of teeth and dental arch form on the Japanese normal occlusion. Shikwa Gakuho 80:945–969

10. Watanabe K, Koga M, Yatabe K, Motegi E, Isshiki Y A 1996 A morphometric study on setup models of Japanese malocclusions. Shikwa Gakuho 96:209–222

11. Trevisi Zanelato A C 2003 Evaluation of dental angulation and tipping in Brazilian subjects presenting natural normal occlusion. Thesis (Master Degree in Orthodontics), Methodist University of São Paulo, Brazil

12. Kalange J T 1999 Ideal appliance placement with APC brackets and indirect bonding. Journal of Clinical Orthodontics 33:516–526

13. Zanelato R C, Grossi A T, Mandetta S, Scanavini M A A 2004 Individualization of torque for the canine teeth in the preadjusted appliance. Revista Clinical Dental Press, Maringa 3:39–54

14. Trevisi H J 2005 The SmartClip self-ligating appliance system. Technique Guide. 3M Company

CHAPTER 3 CLINICAL CASE

Name: N C
Sex: Female
Age: 11.10 years
Facial pattern: Dolichofacial
Skeletal pattern: Class II

Diagnosis

Class I malocclusion with severe upper and lower arch discrepancy and crossbite of upper right lateral incisor (tooth 12).

Treatment plan

The treatment was carried out in two stages:

- In the first stage, a removable appliance was used to correct the upper left lateral incisor crossbite. Subsequently, an upper palatal bar and a lower lingual arch were placed while serial extractions of the deciduous teeth and the first premolars were carried out.

- In the second stage, the anchorage devices (the palatal bar and the lingual arch) were kept in place, and the SmartClip™ Self-Ligating Appliance was used in both upper and lower arches.

Appliance

- Upper palatal bar
- Lower lingual arch
- Upper and lower SmartClip™ Self-Ligating Appliance
- Upper modified Hawley wraparound retainer
- Lower 3–3 fixed retainer

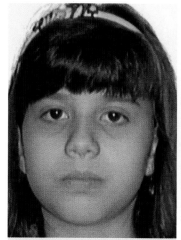 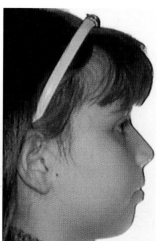

Fig. 3.82   Fig. 3.83

Figs 3.82 & 3.83
Pretreatment photographs showing adequate facial symmetry, facial profile and lip seal.

Case report

The patient presented a severe arch discrepancy in the mixed dentition. Serial extractions of the deciduous teeth and the upper and lower first premolars were carried out to facilitate tooth eruption. To enhance molar anchorage, the palatal bar and the lingual arch were kept in place through the extraction stage until the end of the leveling.

Early in the treatment, .014 and .016 Nitinol round archwires were used, and in the leveling stage .018 and .020 stainless steel round archwires were used. During the space closure stage, .019/.025 stainless steel archwires with hooks prewelded mesial to the canine brackets were used. In the final stage of treatment, .019/.025 rectangular braided archwires were used.

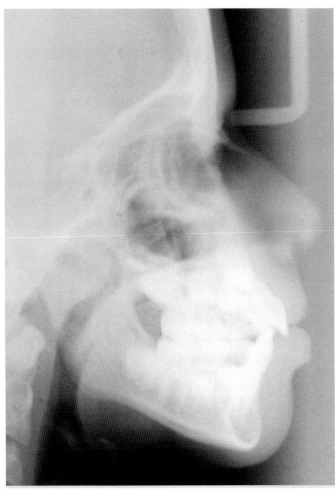

Fig. 3.84

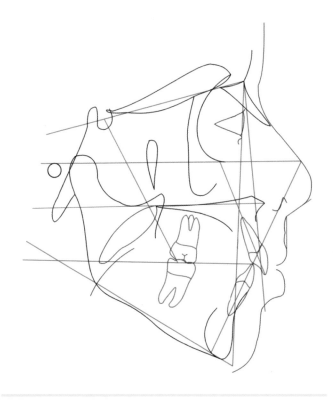

Fig. 3.85

SNA ∠	81°
SNB ∠	73°
ANB ∠	8°
A-N ⊥ FH	5 mm
Po-N ⊥ FH	−5 mm
Wits	8 mm
GoGn SN ∠	43°
FH Md ∠	30°
Mx Md ∠	31°
U1 to A-Po	9 mm
L1 to A-Po	2 mm
U1 to Mx plane ∠	111°
L1 to Md plane ∠	85°
Facial analysis	
Nasolabial ∠	124°
NA ⊥ nose	25 mm
Lip thickness	6 mm

Fig. 3.86

Figs 3.84, 3.85 & 3.86
Cephalometric X-ray, tracing and measurements show well-positioned incisors and a high angle growth pattern.

Figs 3.87, 3.88 & 3.89
Pretreatment intraoral photographs of the mixed dentition, showing crossbite of the upper right lateral incisor, lack of space for the permanent canines and mild Class II malocclusion on the right side.

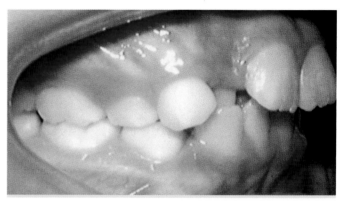

Fig. 3.87

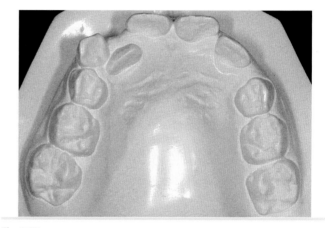

Fig. 3.90

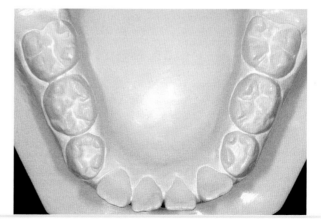

Fig. 3.91

Figs 3.90 & 3.91
Pretreatment study models showing Class I molar relationship and crossbite of the right lateral incisors.

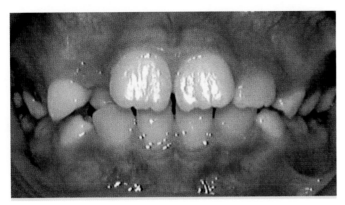

Fig. 3.88

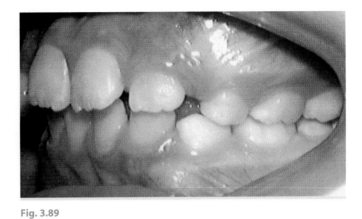

Fig. 3.89

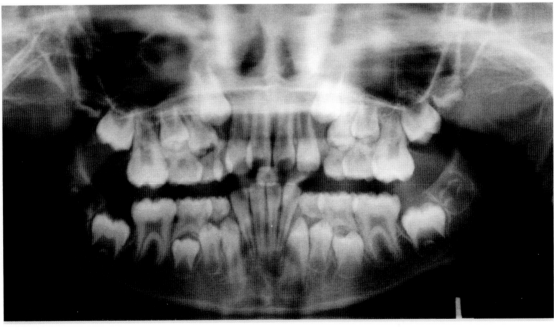

Fig. 3.92

Fig. 3.92
Panoramic X-ray showing normal eruption pattern with severe arch discrepancy and crowding.

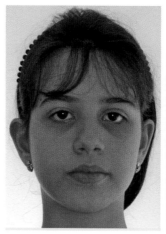 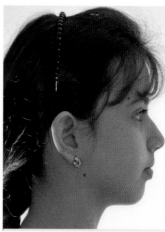

Figs 3.93 & 3.94
Interim photographs showing good facial balance with
adequate lip seal.

Fig. 3.93   Fig. 3.94

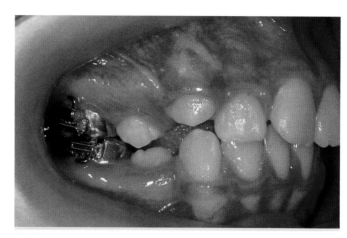

Figs 3.96, 3.97 & 3.98
Intraoral photographs after serial extractions, while
waiting for the eruption of the remaining teeth. Note
the good molar relationship.

Fig. 3.96

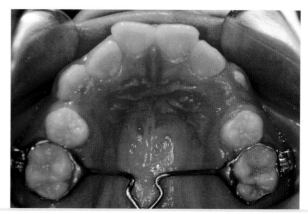

Figs 3.99 & 3.100
Upper and lower occlusal views after the serial
extractions, showing the upper palatal bar, lower
lingual arch and mild discrepancy in the lower arch.

Fig. 3.99

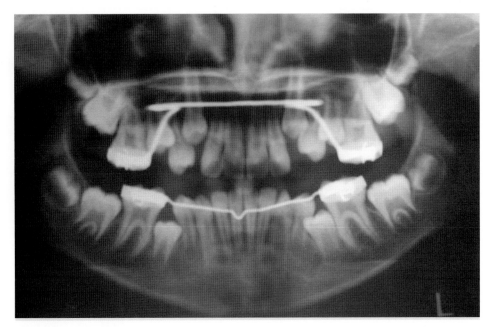

Fig. 3.95
Panoramic X-ray showing normal eruption pattern after extraction of the deciduous teeth.

Fig. 3.95

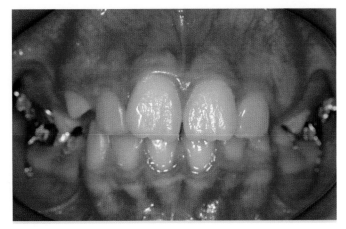

Fig. 3.97

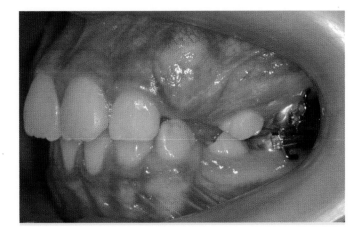

Fig. 3.98

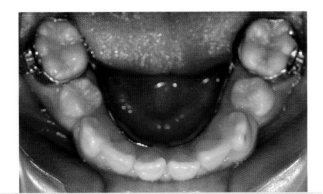

Fig. 3.100

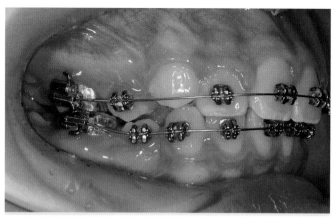

Fig. 3.101

Figs 3.101, 3.102 & 3.103
Partial set-up of the SmartClip™ Self-Ligating
Appliance in the upper and lower arches. Beginning of
the aligning stage with .014 Nitinol archwire.

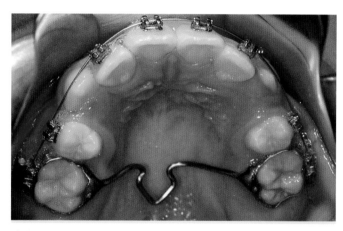

Fig. 3.104

Figs 3.104 & 3.105
Upper and lower occlusal views showing the .014
Nitinol archwires in place at the beginning of the
aligning stage. The palatal bar and the lingual arch
were kept until the end of the aligning stage to
maintain anchorage.

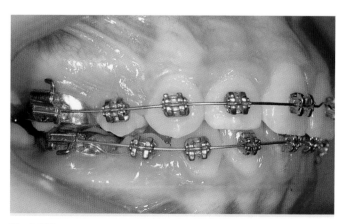

Fig. 3.106

Figs 3.106, 3.107 & 3.108
Upper .016 Nitinol round archwire at the end of the
aligning stage, with brackets placed on the canines.

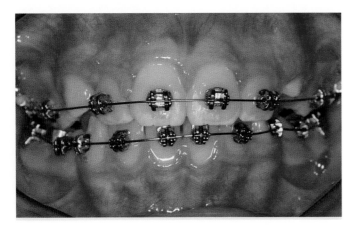

Fig. 3.102

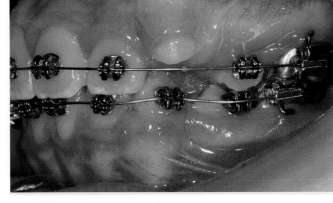

Fig. 3.103

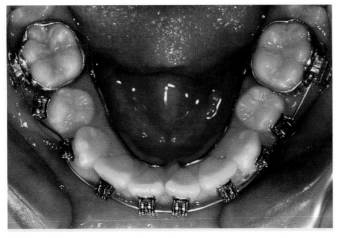

Fig. 3.105

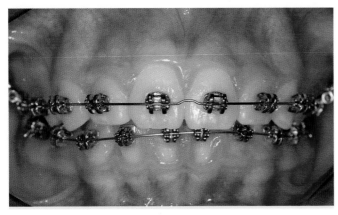

Fig. 3.107

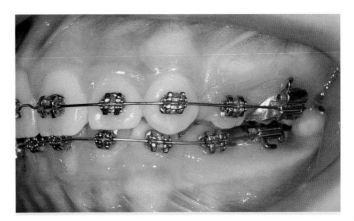

Fig. 3.108

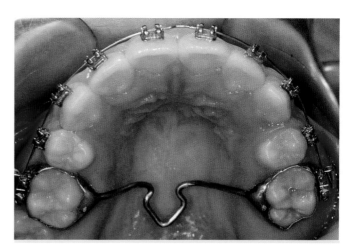

Fig. 3.109

Figs 3.109 & 3.110
Upper and lower occlusal views of the leveling stage with .016 Nitinol round archwire in the upper arch and .016 stainless steel round archwire in the lower arch. The lingual arch has been removed.

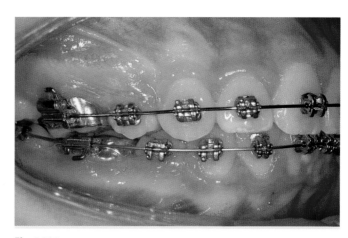

Fig. 3.111

Figs 3.111, 3.112 & 3.113
Upper .020 stainless steel round archwire and lower .018 Nitinol round archwire with bonded tubes on the second molars at the end of the leveling stage.

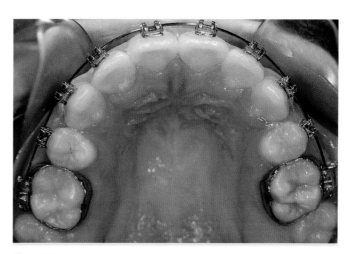

Figs 3.114 & 3.115
Upper and lower occlusal views of the upper .020 stainless steel round archwire, and .018 Nitinol round archwire with bonded tubes on the second molars.

Fig. 3.114

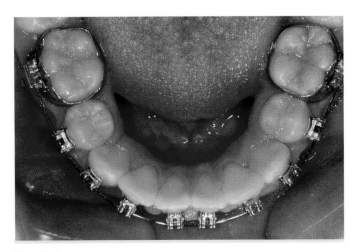

Fig. 3.110

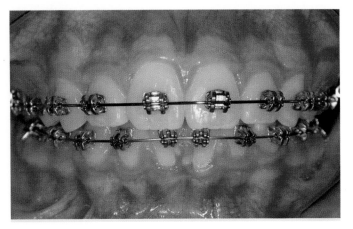

Fig. 3.112

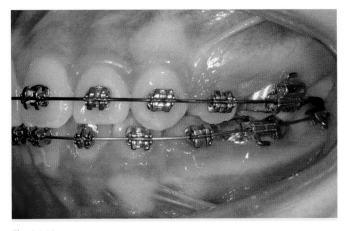

Fig. 3.113

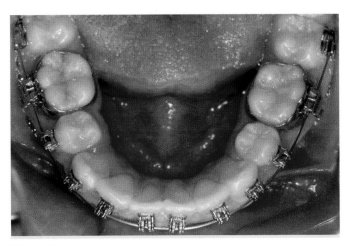

Fig. 3.115

Figs 3.116, 3.117 & 3.118
Upper and lower .019/.025 stainless steel rectangular archwires with prewelded hooks mesial to the canines. In the upper arch, there is a passive laceback on the right side and a tieback on the left side. In the lower arch there are tiebacks on both sides.

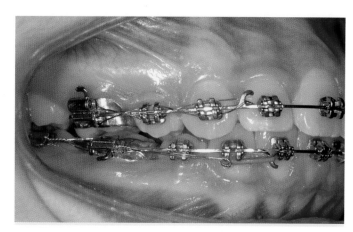

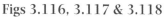
Fig. 3.116

Figs 3.119 & 3.120
Upper and lower occlusal views of the upper and lower .019/.025 stainless steel rectangular archwires during closure of the remaining spaces in the first premolar extraction sites.

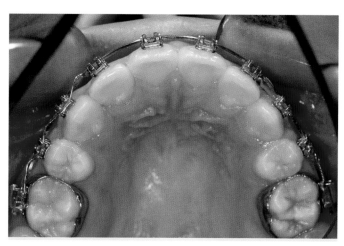

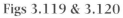
Fig. 3.119

Figs 3.121, 3.122 & 3.123
Upper and lower .019/.025 stainless steel rectangular archwires with prewelded hooks mesial to the canines. Space closure in the extraction sites along with Class II elastics on both sides.

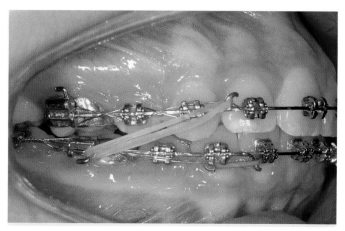

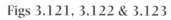
Fig. 3.121

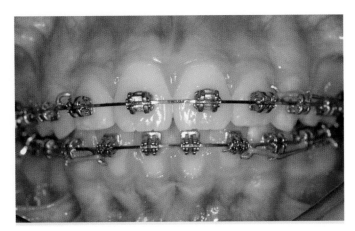

Fig. 3.117

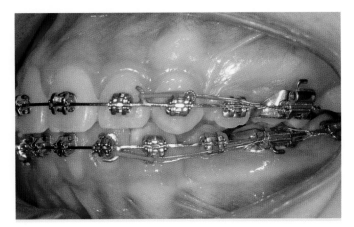

Fig. 3.118

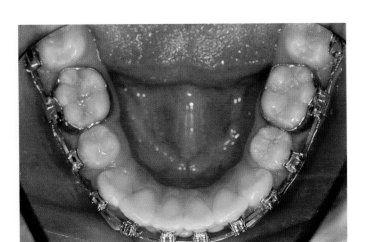

Fig. 3.120

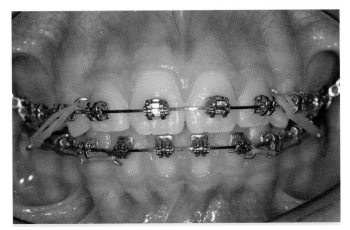

Fig. 3.122

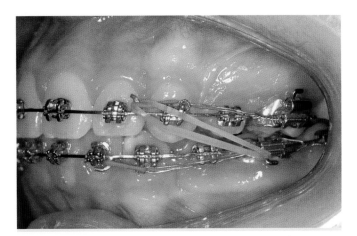

Fig. 3.123

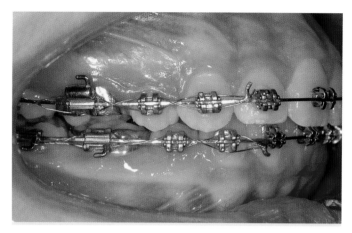

Figs 3.124, 3.125 & 3.126
Upper and lower .019/.025 stainless steel rectangular archwire with prewelded hooks mesial to the canines and passive lacebacks in both arches after space closure. Note the buccal tubes on the upper second molars.

Fig. 3.124

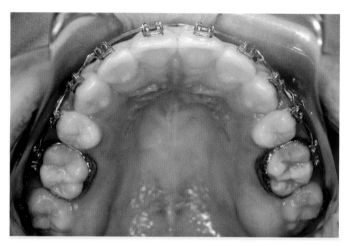

Fig. 3.127

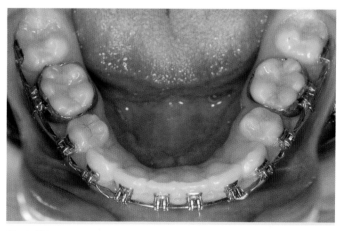

Figs 3.127 & 3.128
Upper and lower occlusal views showing upper and lower arch forms and alignment of teeth with .019/.025 stainless steel rectangular archwires.

Fig. 3.128

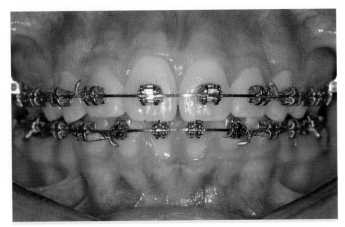

Fig. 3.125

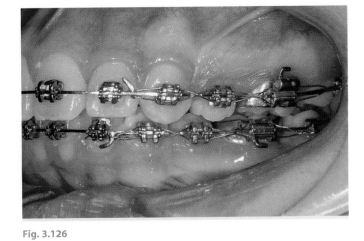

Fig. 3.126

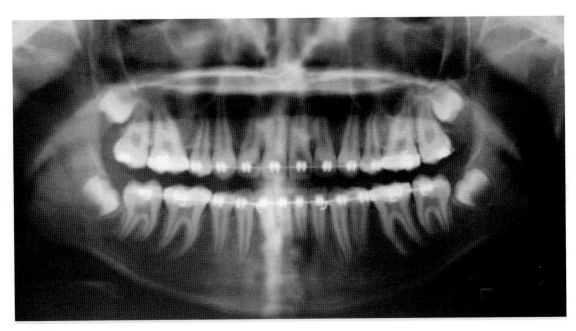

Fig. 3.129

Fig. 3.129
Panoramic X-ray showing dilacerated roots and root parallelism.

Figs 3.130, 3.131 & 3.132
Final stage of treatment with .019/.025 braided archwire in the upper and lower arches for detailing the occlusion.

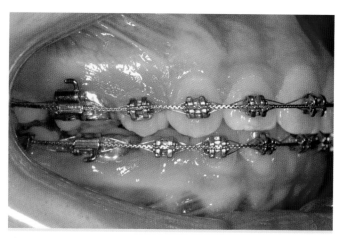

Fig. 3.130

Figs 3.133, 3.134 & 3.135
Detailing the occlusion with .019/.025 rectangular braided archwire in both arches. Note the finishing elastics on the premolars and molars.

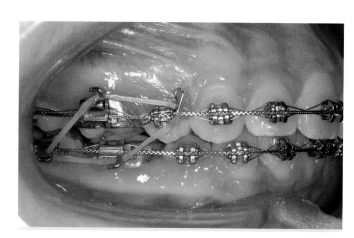

Fig. 3.133

Figs 3.136, 3.137 & 3.138
Final view of the occlusion after use of the finishing elastics. Both arches have the .019/.025 braided archwires.

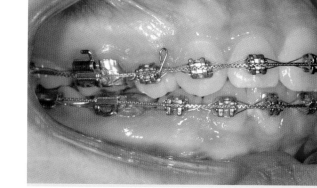

Fig. 3.136

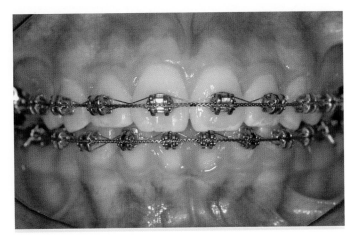

Fig. 3.131

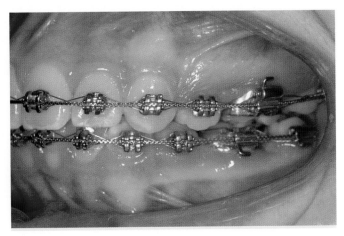

Fig. 3.132

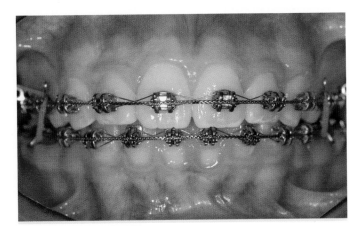

Fig. 3.134

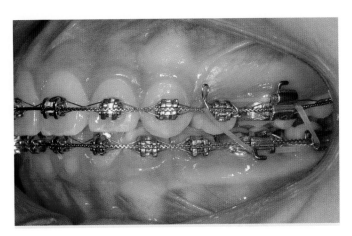

Fig. 3.135

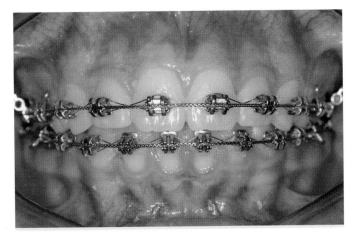

Fig. 3.137

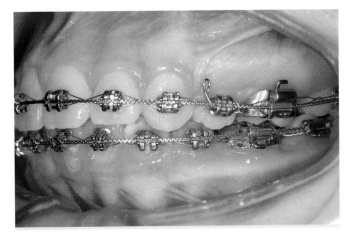

Fig. 3.138

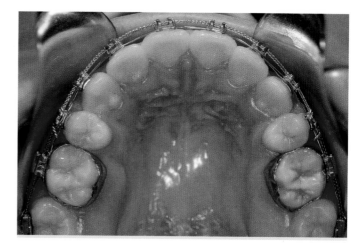

Fig. 3.139

Figs 3.139, 3.140 & 3.141
Upper and lower occlusal views showing the arch forms, alignment and points of contact between the teeth. Anterior guidance achieved at the end of the orthodontic treatment.

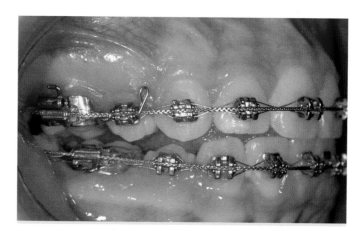

Fig. 3.142

Figs 3.142, 3.143 & 3.144
Checking the functional movements before appliance removal. Note the posterior disclusion due to the incisor guidance with adequate interocclusal space in the molars and premolars area.

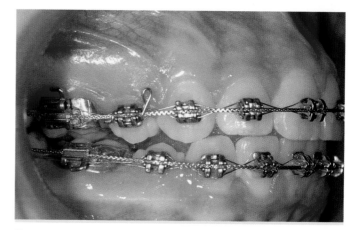

Fig. 3.145

Figs 3.145, 3.146 & 3.147
Checking the functional movements. Lateroprotrusive disclusion on the right side due to the canine guidance (mutually protected occlusion) with adequate interocclusal space on both working and non-working sides.

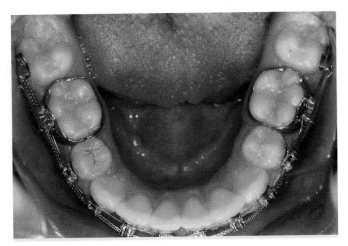

Fig. 3.140

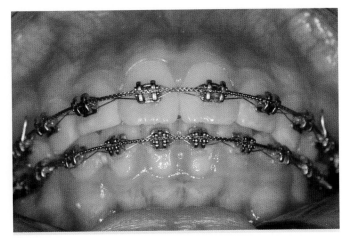

Fig. 3.141

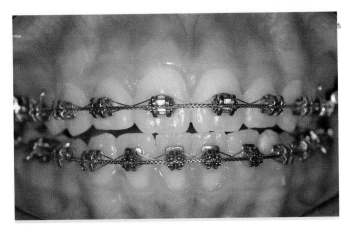

Fig. 3.143

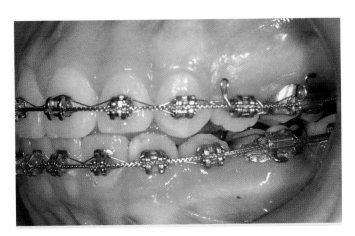

Fig. 3.144

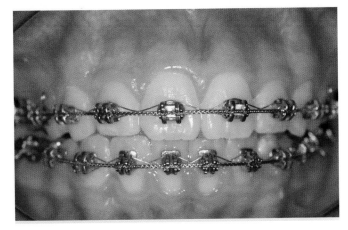

Fig. 3.146

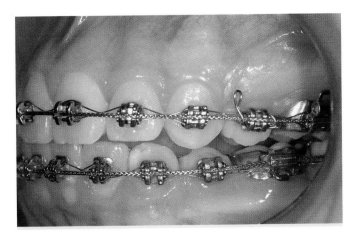

Fig. 3.147

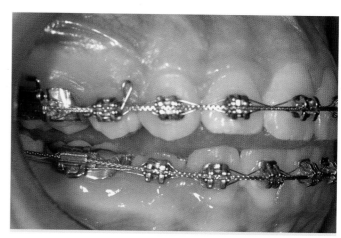

Figs 3.148, 3.149 & 3.150
Checking the functional movements. Lateroprotrusive disclusion on the left side due to the canine guidance (mutually protected occlusion) with adequate interocclusal space on both working and non-working sides.

Fig. 3.148

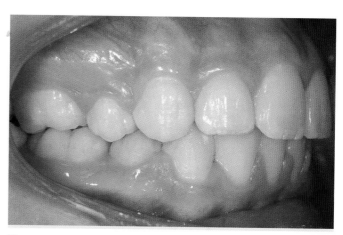

Figs 3.151, 3.152 & 3.153
Post-treatment photographs showing maximum intercuspation.

Fig. 3.151

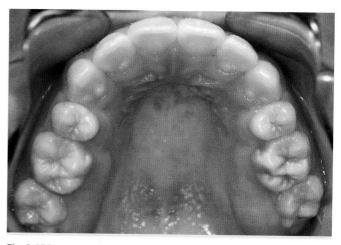

Figs 3.154, 3.155 & 3.156
Post-treatment upper and lower occlusal views showing a good arch form, alignment and points of contact between the teeth. Anterior guidance and overbite providing good functional movements.

Fig. 3.154

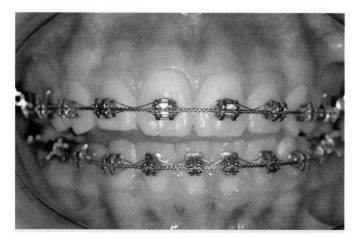

Fig. 3.149

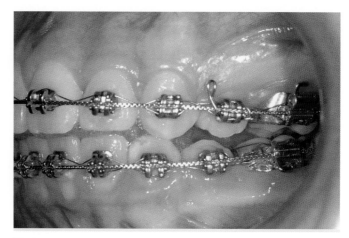

Fig. 3.150

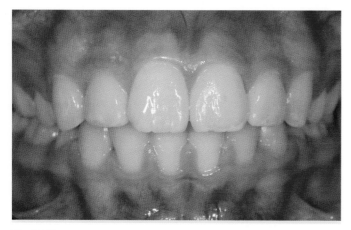

Fig. 3.152

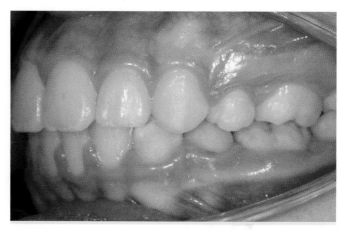

Fig. 3.153

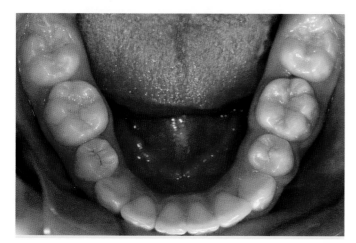

Fig. 3.155

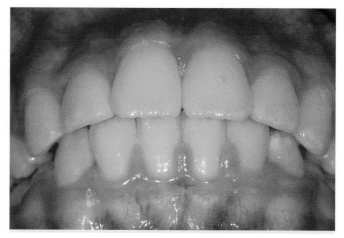

Fig. 3.156

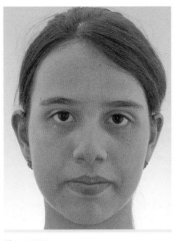

Fig. 3.157

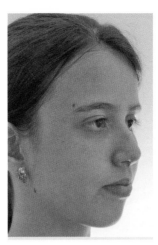

Fig. 3.158

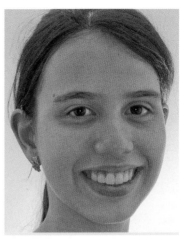

Fig. 3.159

Fig. 3.160

Figs 3.157 & 3.158
Post-treatment photographs showing good facial balance.

Figs 3.159 & 3.160
Post-treatment three-quarter and smiling photographs showing good facial balance and smile line.

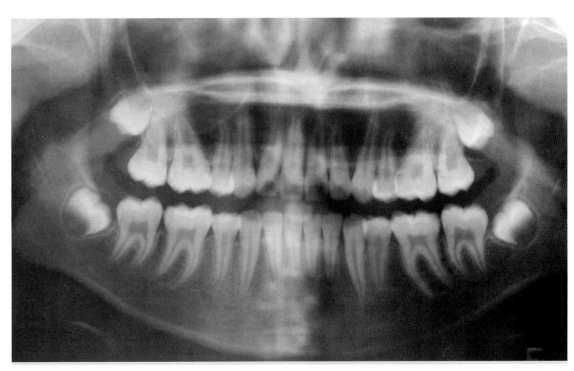

Fig. 3.161

Fig. 3.161
Post-treatment panoramic X-ray showing root dilaceration and parallelism between the roots.

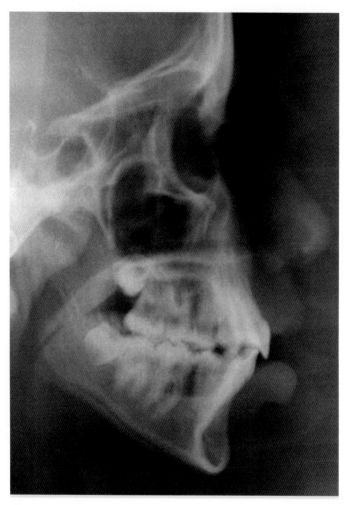

Fig. 3.162

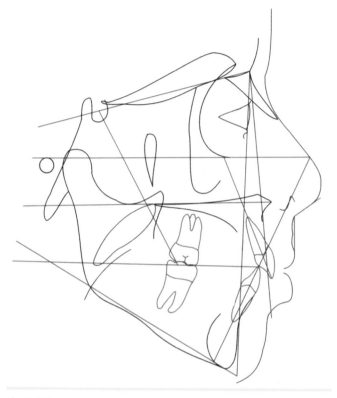

Fig. 3.163

SNA ∠	84°
SNB ∠	76°
ANB ∠	8°
A-N ⊥ FH	6 mm
Po-N ⊥ FH	−2 mm
Wits	2 mm
GoGn SN ∠	44°
FH Md ∠	33°
Mx Md ∠	36°
U1 to A-Po	8 mm
L1 to A-Po	5 mm
U1 to Mx plane ∠	108°
L1 to Md plane ∠	94°
Facial analysis	
Nasolabial ∠	105°
NA ⊥ nose	29 mm
Lip thickness	9 mm

Figs 3.162, 3.163 & 3.164
Post-treatment cephalometric X-ray, tracing and measurements.

Fig. 3.164

Sliding mechanics for orthodontic movements

Introduction

With the development of the Straight-Wire™ Appliance[1] in the early 1970s, the first, second and third order bends were built individually into each bracket for both the upper and lower arches. To avoid putting any bends in the archwire, Andrews envisaged that different totally programmed brackets would need to be used, depending on the patient's malocclusion and the magnitude of tooth movement. However, the concept of using totally programmed brackets requires the clinician to have a large inventory of brackets available in the clinic and was a major barrier to the development of this first generation of programmed appliances.

In 1975, Roth, who was following Andrews' concept of using a .021/.025 rectangular stainless steel archwire in a .022/.028 slot for space closure and in the final stage of treatment, tried to solve the inventory problem.[2] Roth favored an appliance system with a minimum number of brackets that, according to him, could be used in both extraction and non-extraction cases. This led to a major reformulation of the original prescription of the Straight-Wire™ Appliance (the second generation of preadusted appliances) and substantial improvement in the straight-wire technique.

Since then, the Straight-Wire™ Appliance has been the subject of much research aimed at evaluating the data collected by Andrews, with the additional goals of improving the appliance prescription, simplifying the mechanics and reducing the need for adding bends to orthodontic archwires. Nonetheless, the treatment goals continue to be the same – establishing correct positioning of teeth at the end of the orthodontic treatment to obtain functional balance and stable results. Thus studies have also been evaluating the correct angulation and inclination of teeth, using as a reference the tooth positions in individuals with normal occlusion.

In 1997, to overcome the inadequacies of the original Straight-Wire™ Appliance, McLaughlin, Bennett and Trevisi worked together to design a new bracket system.[3] These authors reviewed Andrews' research[1] and compared the data with the results of Japanese studies.[4,5] This research triggered the development of the MBT™ Appliance System – the third generation of preadjusted appliances. The MBT™ Appliance System introduced improvements and modifications to the bracket prescription to solve clinical problems, based on a balance between science and 25 years of clinical experience of the three authors. It features rhomboidal-shaped brackets and a prescription compatible with sliding mechanics and the use of a .019/.025 archwire in the .022/.028 slot during space closure.[3,6]

Sliding mechanics

Before developing the MBT™ Appliance, McLaughlin, Bennett and Trevisi worked with several different prescriptions of brackets. This experience helped in designing the MBT™ Appliance to meet the new concept of sliding mechanics and light forces. It is the force levels and the mechanics that determine the features of the orthodontic appliance, and not vice versa. These factors also determine the tooth movements during the three stages of orthodontic treatment – aligning, leveling and space closure. During aligning and leveling, the teeth slide on the archwire, whereas, during space closure, the archwire slides through the slots of the brackets and the buccal tubes (Figs 4.1 & 4.2). Throughout the treatment the clinician needs to pay close attention to undesired tooth movement. Better results are achieved with sliding mechanics when there is reduced friction between the bracket slot and the archwire, and when low force levels are applied.[3]

SmartClip™ Self-Ligating Appliance

The main advantage of the SmartClip™ Self-Ligating Appliance[7] is the reduced friction between the bracket slot and the archwire, which decreases force levels and facilitates the principles of sliding mechanics, e.g.

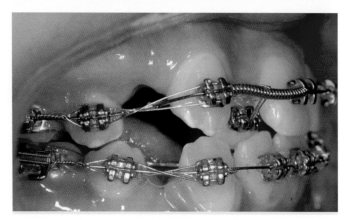

Fig. 4.1 Beginning of the aligning stage: sliding mechanics on a .014 rounded Nitinol archwire. Individual retraction of the canine with a metal ligature to relieve the crowding (the tooth slides on the wire).

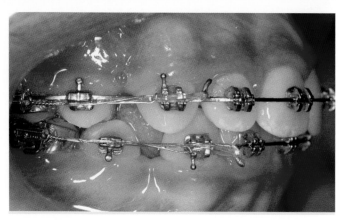

Fig. 4.2 During space closure, metal ligatures are used along with elastic modules. Note the .019/.025 rectangular stainless steel archwire (archwire slides through the bracket slot) and buccal tubes on the posterior teeth.

using the .022/.028 slot and a .019/.025 rectangular archwire during the final stages of orthodontic treatment. Orthodontic treatment using the SmartClip™ Self-Ligating Appliance is completed using a .019/.025 archwire. This archwire allows good sliding mechanics and adequate three-dimensional control of teeth in the anterior and posterior segments of both arches.

Friction, which is typically established between the orthodontic archwire and the bracket slot by the elastic and metal ligatures, prevents ideal movement of teeth during orthodontic treatment. With the SmartClip™ Self-Ligating Appliance, ligatures are not used because the archwire is held in the bracket slot by the lateral clips, allowing free movement of the teeth.

Anchorage control

The choice of anchorage during the orthodontic treatment is very important. The anchorage needs should be defined at the beginning of treatment, and good management of anchorage will lead to good clinical results. Comprehension and control of the reaction forces to the orthodontic forces, including undesirable tooth movement, can make a difference to the clinical results. Anchorage needs vary from case to case and should be based on the discrepancy present in both arches. For example, if there is severe protrusion

and/or anterior crowding, the posterior teeth will require greater mesial control. There are three systems of anchorage that may be used during orthodontic treatment: reciprocal anchorage, moderate anchorage and maximum anchorage.

Reciprocal anchorage is an adequate option for most treatments involving extraction of premolars.[3] This system provides more freedom of movement for the posterior teeth. Zanelato evaluated the loss of anchorage with regard to the lower first molars in cases treated with extractions of the first and second premolars with the straight-wire technique,[8] and found that about 50% of the existing space is closed by the mesial movement of the posterior teeth, whereas the other 50% is closed by the distal movement of the anterior teeth. With the use of SmartClip™ Self-Ligating Appliance System, there is no need to use additional anchorage devices because teeth move freely. Mesial movement of posterior teeth can help provide space for the eruption of third molars, thus establishing a final occlusion with 28 teeth. This is a positive outcome, as most orthodontic treatments involving premolar extractions[8] and anchorage control leave an occlusion with 24 teeth due to lack of space in the posterior regions of the dental arches.

Usually reciprocal anchorage is used in orthodontic treatment with premolar extractions in two clinical situations:

● when the lower first premolars are extracted and buccal tubes are placed on the first molars

● when the second premolars are extracted and the appliance set-up includes the second molars.

With reciprocal anchorage the orthodontic movements in the anterior and posterior segments will be close to reciprocity, that is, 3.5 mm of tooth movement in the anterior segment, and 3.5 mm of tooth movement in

the posterior segment (assuming the premolars measure 7 mm) (Figs 4.3, 4.4 & 4.5).

Moderate anchorage is used when the total discrepancy in the lower arch is between 8 mm and 10 mm. In these situations, 25% of the extraction spaces are closed by the mesial movement of the posterior teeth and 75% by the distal movement of the anterior teeth. The movement of the posterior teeth is controlled by appliances that preserve anchorage, such

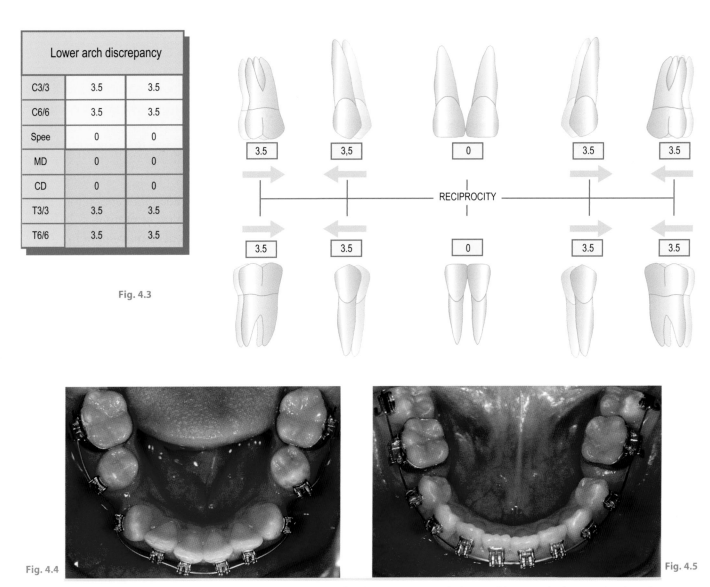

Lower arch discrepancy		
C3/3	3.5	3.5
C6/6	3.5	3.5
Spee	0	0
MD	0	0
CD	0	0
T3/3	3.5	3.5
T6/6	3.5	3.5

Fig. 4.3

Fig. 4.4

Fig. 4.5

Figs 4.3, 4.4 & 4.5   Simulation of movement using the reciprocal anchorage system, in which 50% of the spaces in the extraction sites of first and second premolars are closed by the anterior teeth and 50% by the posterior teeth. Fig. 4.4: A case with extraction of the first premolars and anchorage involving only the first molars. Fig. 4.5: A case with extraction of the second premolars with anchorage involving the second molars as well. MD, midline; CD, cephalometric discrepancy.

as a palatal bar in the upper arch, and a lingual arch in the lower arch.[3] Generally, anchorage devices should remain in place until the end of leveling. Another recommendation is to include the second molars in the appliance set-up. These teeth provide additional anchorage due to their great radicular mass and their location, which is in an area of great bone density in the mandible (Figs 4.6, 4.7, 4.8 & 4.9).

Lower arch discrepancy		
C3/3	5	5
C6/6	5	5
Spee	0	0
MD	0	0
CD	0	0
T3/3	5	5
T6/6	5	5

Fig. 4.6

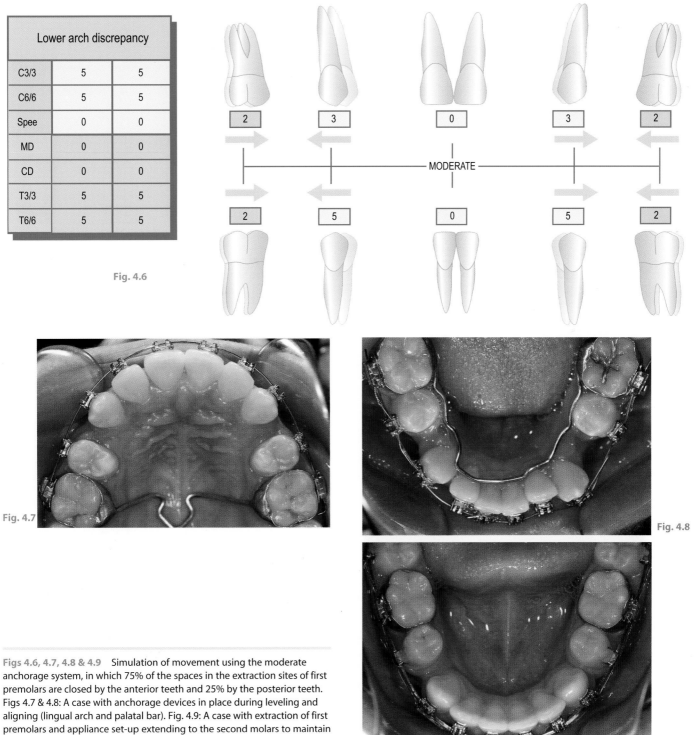

Figs 4.6, 4.7, 4.8 & 4.9 Simulation of movement using the moderate anchorage system, in which 75% of the spaces in the extraction sites of first premolars are closed by the anterior teeth and 25% by the posterior teeth. Figs 4.7 & 4.8: A case with anchorage devices in place during leveling and aligning (lingual arch and palatal bar). Fig. 4.9: A case with extraction of first premolars and appliance set-up extending to the second molars to maintain anchorage. MD, midline; CD, cephalometric discrepancy.

Fig. 4.7

Fig. 4.8

Fig. 4.9

The maximum anchorage system is used when the total discrepancy in the dental arches is between 10 mm and 14 mm. In these clinical cases, there is often severe anterior crowding and dental protrusion, and the extraction spaces are closed by just the distal movement of the anterior teeth due to the severity of the anterior discrepancy. Anchorage devices should be inserted **prior to** the extractions to avoid any mesial movement of the posterior teeth. They should remain in place throughout treatment (Figs 4.10, 4.11 & 4.12). Currently, orthodontic mini-implants are being used in maximum anchorage cases to provide absolute anchorage. These can be used for several purposes, and are thus becoming an essential tool in complex orthodontic cases (Fig. 4.13).

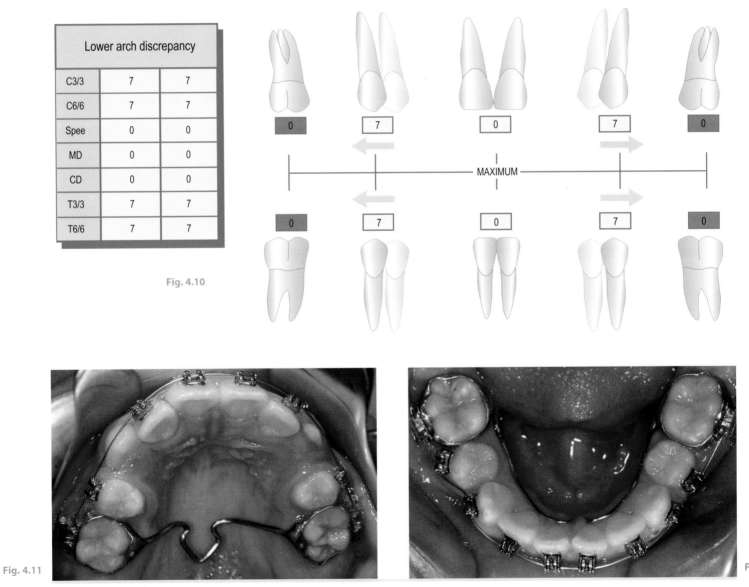

Lower arch discrepancy		
C3/3	7	7
C6/6	7	7
Spee	0	0
MD	0	0
CD	0	0
T3/3	7	7
T6/6	7	7

Fig. 4.10

Fig. 4.11

Fig. 4.12

Figs 4.10, 4.11 & 4.12 Simulation of movement using the maximum anchorage system, in which the spaces from the extraction site of first premolars are occupied by the anterior teeth. In maximum anchorage cases, anchorage devices should be used throughout the treatment. MD, midline; CD, cephalometric discrepancy.

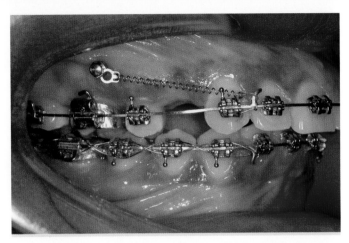

Fig. 4.13   Case requiring maximum anchorage. Upper first premolars were extracted and mini-implants placed. The case was finished in a Class II molar relationship.

Archwire sequencing

The essence of the SmartClip™ Self-Ligating Appliance System is the perfect combination of the mechanics and the orthodontic archwire during all stages of the orthodontic treatment. The archwire is held in the bracket slot by two clips located on the mesial and distal wings of the bracket.[7] This allows free movement of the teeth when applying sliding mechanics.

The SmartClip™ Self-Ligating Appliance is classified as a **passive appliance**, because the archwire retention system does not put any pressure on the archwire in the bracket slot. The archwire works freely within the bracket slot, and, accordingly, rotations should be corrected in the early stages of the treatment. The archwire sequence should be based on correcting rotations during the beginning of aligning. Thinner rectangular Nitinol archwires should be used at the end of the aligning stage.

The following archwire sequence is recommended[7] for the aligning, leveling, space closure and finishing stages of treatment:

Aligning

.014 classic Nitinol archwire or .014 superelastic Nitinol

.016 classic Nitinol archwire or .016 superelastic Nitinol

.016/.025 classic Nitinol archwire or .016/.025 superelastic Nitinol

.017/.025 classic Nitinol archwire or .017/.025 superelastic Nitinol

Leveling

.019/.025 classic Nitinol archwire or .019/.025 superelastic Nitinol

.019/.025 classic Nitinol-Hybrid

.021/.025 Nitinol superelastic-Hybrid

Space closure

.019/.025 stainless steel archwire

Finishing and detailing

.019/.025 braided archwire

Aligning

Aligning is the first stage of orthodontic treatment, and the goal is to obtain space to correct crowding and rotations, reestablish the contact points of teeth and initiate the process of achieving an ideal arch form for the patient.

The author recommends using the .022/.028 bracket slot. Alignment should start with .014 or .016 round classic or superelastic Nitinol archwires, depending on crowding and the severity of the initial malocclusion. These archwires work more freely within the bracket slot. In this first stage of treatment, adequate space should be made to correct crowding, especially in premolar extraction cases (Figs 4.14 & 4.15). After initial alignment, the round archwires should be replaced by .016/.025 or .017/.025 rectangular classic or superelastic Nitinol archwires to correct rotations in cases with and without extractions (Figs 4.16, 4.17 & 4.18).

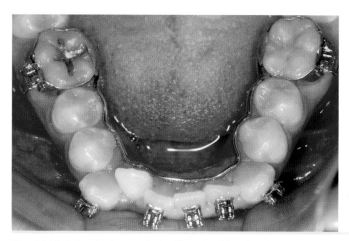
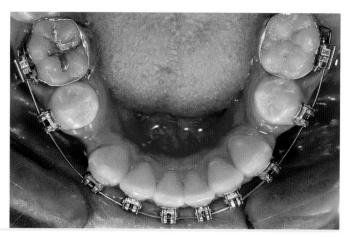

Figs 4.14 & 4.15   Anchorage device (lingual arch) and appliance set-up (SmartClip™ Self-Ligating Appliance) on the lower arch before doing the extractions. Aligning is finalized after distalization of the canines on a .014 round Nitinol archwire.

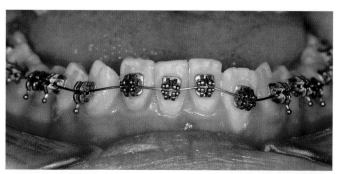

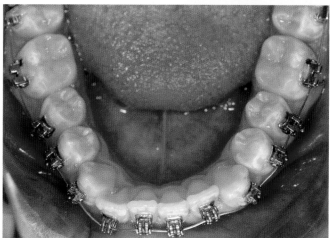
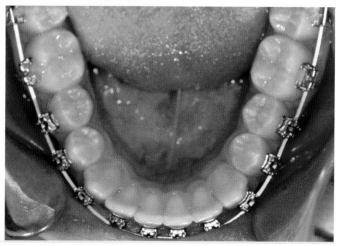

Figs 4.16, 4.17 & 4.18   Initial stage of non-extraction treatment: .014 round Nitinol archwire engaged. Finalizing aligning: .017/.025 rectangular Nitinol archwire engaged. Rotations and contact points have been corrected.

Lacebacks

In the early 1970s, the Straight-Wire Appliance[1] prescription incorporated excessive angulation for the anterior teeth. Thus during aligning and leveling, there was a tendency for protrusion of the canines and the incisors, as well as increase in anterior overbite and openbites in the premolar region. Concern about these adverse effects prompted the developers of the MBT™ treatment philosophy to develop mechanics to overcome such setbacks. The lacebacks from molars to canines were found to minimize the undesired movements, and avoid the mesial tipping of the canine crowns,[3] thus allowing their roots to move distally. It was seen that the lacebacks also allowed the distal movement of the canines, resulting in the treatment of anterior crowding in a coordinated and balanced way (Figs 4.19 & 4.20). Later, as appliances incorporating reduced angulation for the anterior teeth became available for the anterior teeth, such problems almost disappeared. However, lacebacks continue to be used for sliding mechanics, aimed at distal movement of the canines. The .009 metal ligature is recommended for use during sliding mechanics.

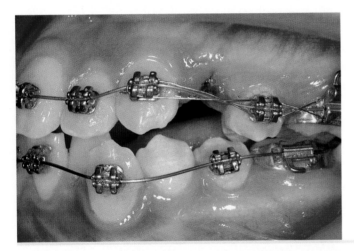
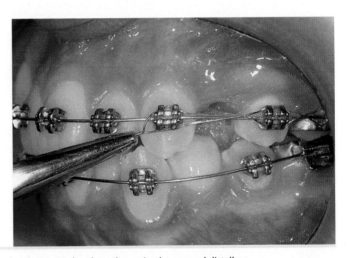

Figs 4.19 & 4.20   Laceback being put at the beginning of aligning on a .014 round archwire; 30 days later the canine has moved distally.

Leveling

After finishing aligning with a .016/.025 or .017/.025 Nitinol archwire, a .019/.025 rectangular classic Nitinol, superelastic or hybrid, or .021/.025 rectangular hybrid archwire should be used during the leveling stage. At this stage of treatment, all the teeth should be included in the set-up (Figs 4.21, 4.22 & 4.23).

During leveling, the clinician should evaluate the overbite and the curve of Spee,[9] as well as the need to start correcting these before commencing with the space closure stage of treatment. If there is a severe overbite and deep curve of Spee, the second molars should be included in the treatment as soon as possible and .018 and .020 stainless steel archwires used (Fig. 4.24).[3] These archwires should remain in place for a longer period, allowing them to correct the overbite and curve of Spee.

Leveling is the preparatory stage for space closure, and therefore it should be well executed. At this stage, check the positioning of brackets and buccal tubes and rebond where necessary. The main points that should be checked before finishing leveling are:

- reestablishment of the contact points
- correction of the rotations
- correction of the angulations

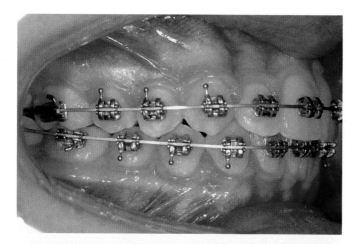

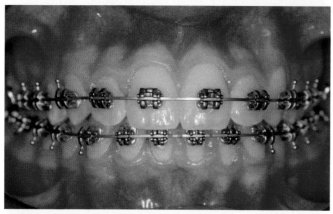

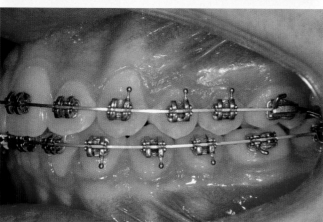

Figs 4.21, 4.22 & 4.23 Upper and lower .019/.025 rectangular classic Nitinol archwires finalizing leveling.

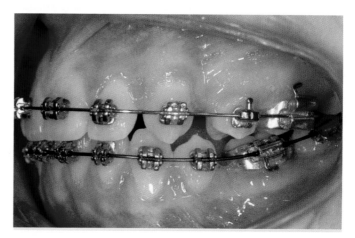

Fig. 4.24 In deep overbite cases, buccal tubes should be bonded on the lower second molars and .018 and .020 round stainless steel archwires should be used to facilitate the correction of the curve of Spee and the overbite.

- alignment of the slots
- correction of the overbite
- leveling of the curve of Spee.

Once all of these have been verified and corrected, space closure can be started.

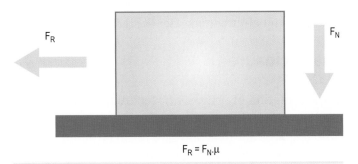

$$F_R = F_N \cdot \mu$$

Fig. 4.25 Friction is generated when two bodies are in contact and slide on one another. The classic friction equation is: product of the normal force between the two bodies and the friction coefficient.

Friction

Friction is generated when two bodies in contact slide on one another (Fig. 4.25). In orthodontics, friction occurs between the bracket slots and the orthodontic archwire when teeth angulation or inclination is not correct or when teeth are rotated. Friction also occurs due to unfinished leveling, or pressure from metal or elastic ligatures and attachments. These factors prevent, or make more difficult, the sliding of the bracket along the archwire and vice versa, increasing the force levels needed and the treatment time.

Friction is influenced by the type, size and material of brackets and archwires, and it occurs regardless of whether the conventional and self-ligating orthodontic technique is used. Three different types of frictional forces occur during orthodontic mechanics: classic friction, binding and notching (Fig. 4.26).

Classic friction

Classic friction results from the use of metal and elastic ligatures when working with conventional appliances. The ligatures keep the archwire engaged in the bracket

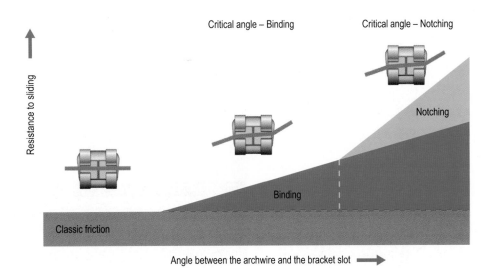

Figs 4.26 Graph showing the types of friction generated when applying orthodontic mechanics – classic friction, binding and notching. Resistance to sliding is generated between the archwire and the bracket slot.

slot, but increase friction. The SmartClip™ Self-Ligating Appliance is associated with very low levels of classic friction because there is no need for ligatures. This in turn allows a reduction in the force levels used during orthodontic treatment with full expression of the bracket prescription and provides more biocompatible tooth movement. When using ligatures with orthodontic appliances, most of the force applied is used to overcome classic friction (Fig. 4.27).

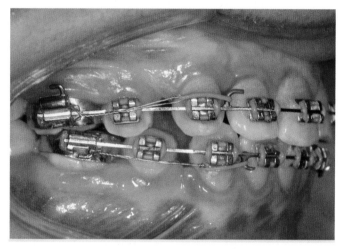

Fig. 4.27 Space closure with sliding mechanics using ligatures. Classic friction is generated by the elastic ligatures.

Binding

Binding occurs in both conventional appliances and self-ligating appliances, and results from the presence of incorrect tooth angulation or inclination rotation or from unfinished leveling. When these factors are not eliminated, resistance is established between the bracket slot and the archwire (Figs 4.28 & 4.29), thus causing binding.

Notching

Notching occurs if there is deformation of the orthodontic archwire during any stage of treatment. This type of friction prevents final correction of rotations and angulations (Figs 4.30 & 4.31).

Space closure

In the evolution of orthodontic techniques, sliding mechanics have been shown to be most effective in closing spaces at extraction sites during treatment with preadjusted appliances. Sliding mechanics involve sliding of rectangular archwires in the bracket slots of premolars and the buccal tubes of molars to close the remaining spaces in the extraction sites (Fig. 4.32).[3]

When the SmartClip™ Self-Ligating Appliance is used, the friction generated by the metal and elastic ligatures

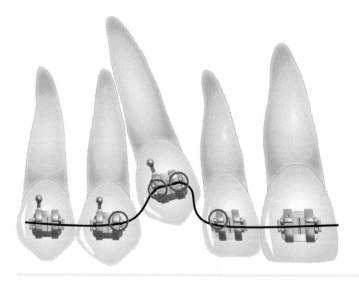

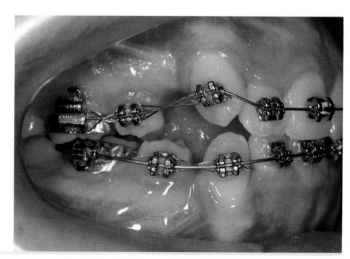

Figs 4.28 & 4.29 Binding (friction) occurs in the distal or mesial part of the bracket between the archwire and the bracket slot.

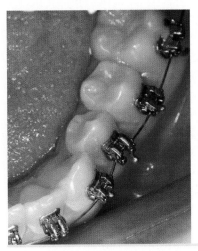

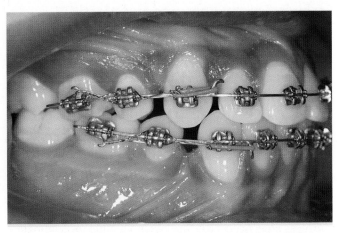

Fig. 4.32   Sliding mechanics with the SmartClip™ Self-Ligating Appliance and a .019/.025 archwire. Note the hook prewelded on the archwire mesial to the canine bracket and use of AlastiK™ modules and metal ligatures.

Figs 4.30 & 4.31   Notching occurs when there is deformation of the orthodontic archwire. Archwire deformation at the mesial side of the left lower first premolar, preventing the correction of the rotation. Archwire after disengagement showing alteration in form.

– classic friction – is eliminated, thus reducing the forces needed during treatment. Figure 4.33 is an example of tooth movement without classic friction as no metal or elastic ligatures have been used. In addition, the SmartClip™ Appliance features reduced angulation for upper and lower anterior teeth, making

aligning and leveling mechanics more efficient by preventing the unwanted effects mentioned above.

The space closure mechanics presented in this chapter are based on several years of experience of the author and its application over a long period of time. This system provides excellent force levels, resulting in tooth movement with good control of the treatment mechanics when closing spaces in the extraction sites. Depending on the magnitude of the overbite and the need for torque control, space closure can be carried out using .019/.025 rectangular stainless steel or Nitinol archwires in .022/.028 slot brackets.

During orthodontic treatment, forces capable of stimulating cellular activity should be applied to maximize tooth movement. Thus, the aim is to have an appliance system that features passive self-ligating brackets and allows the use of high-technology archwires, carefully selected to deliver the optimum force levels during the aligning, leveling and space closure.

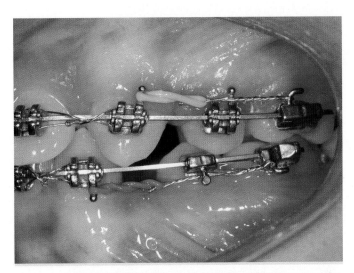

Fig. 4.33   SmartClip™ Self-Ligating Appliance with a .019/.025 rectangular Nitinol archwire with no classic friction established by the use of elastic and metal ligatures during space closure.

Space closure with a .019/.025 stainless steel archwire, metal ligatures and AlastiK™ modules

When using sliding mechanics with a .019/.025 rectangular stainless steel archwire, the .7 mm brass hooks should be welded mesial to the canines (or could be prewelded).[3] To weld the hook, the clinician should precisely mark the point of contact between the canine and lateral incisor, using a Mathieu needle holder to hold the rectangular archwire. The procedure is very simple and allows adequate welding without losing the properties of the archwire (Fig. 4.34). Rectangular stainless steel archwires are also available with hooks prewelded at three different widths between the canines. Thus, the clinician can choose the archwire that best suits the case (Fig. 4.35).

The retraction system comprises a .009 metal ligature tied to an AlastiK™ module. The metal ligature is tied to the molars and then to the AlastiK™ module which is slipped on the hook welded on the stainless steel archwire, mesial to the canine[3] (Figs 4.36, 4.37 & 4.38). The AlastiK™ module should be activated 3 mm or twice the length of the unstretched module (Fig. 4.39). The retraction system should remain in place for

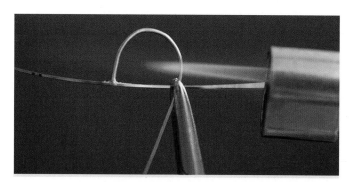

Fig. 4.34 A 0.7 mm brass wire being welded on a .019/.025 archwire. A Mathieu needle holder is used to hold the wires.

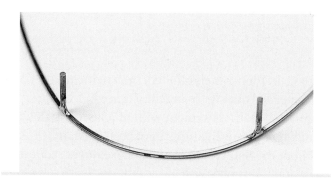

Fig. 4.35 Rectangular archwire with prewelded hooks.

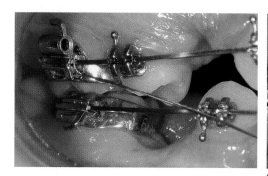

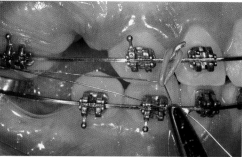

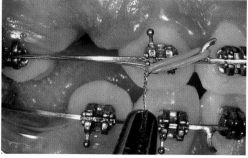

Figs 4.36, 4.37 & 4.38 Metal ligature on the first molar and AlastiK™ module placed on the hook welded to the mesial of the canine. Activate the AlastiK™ module by 3 mm or twice its unstretched length.

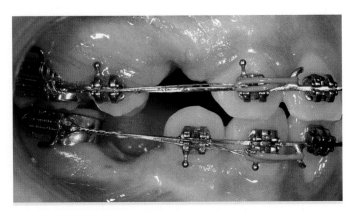

Fig. 4.39 Activation of the retraction system by 3 mm.

30 days, after which it can be replaced or reactivated. The second activation should be twice the length of the AlastiK™ module or until the clinician feels some resistance during the activation. The retraction system should remain in place for another 30 days.

In 2004, Moresca and Vigorito[10] evaluated in vitro the force degradation in elastic modules used to close spaces. They studied the force levels produced at 3 mm and 2 mm activation by four different commercial brands of elastic modules, and verified the degradation of force over a 28-day period. The forces were

measured at six time intervals: initial, 24 hours, 7 days, 14 days, 21 days and 28 days. The study showed that an average force of 193 g was delivered by the 3 mm AlastiK™ module after 24 hours to 28 days, whereas the 2 mm AlastiK™ module delivered 162 g of force (Fig. 4.40).

When the second molar is included in the set-up, the wire ligature should be tied to the hook on the second molar buccal tube to increase the level of activation.

Space closure with a .019/.025 stainless steel archwire and Nitinol springs

The sliding mechanics to close spaces using a rectangular stainless steel archwire can also be applied using Nitinol springs, with the spring placed in a similar way to the AlastiK™ module. First the spring is attached to the hook on the first molar and then onto the hook welded to the archwire mesial to the canine (Fig. 4.41). Springs provide better control of the forces applied and continuous force throughout the time it is in place. Using this system, the interval between appointments can be more than 30 days. If the second molar is included in the set-up, tie the second molar to the first molar with a metal ligature.

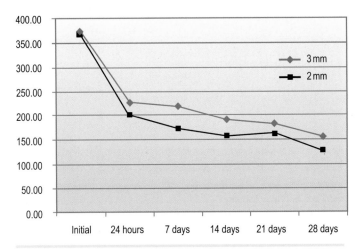

Fig. 4.40 Average force levels (g) generated by elastic modules (3M Unitek) with 3 mm and 2 mm activations in the time intervals studied.

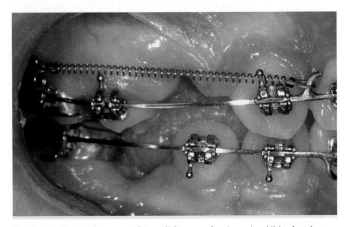

Fig. 4.41 Space closure applying sliding mechanics using Nitinol springs. The clinician needs to pay closer attention to the force level generated by this retraction system.

Space closure with a .019/.025 Nitinol archwire

Retraction with laceback and AlastiK™ modules

The SmartClip™ Self-Ligating Appliance System allows the use of Nitinol archwires during space closure, but there are some issues that should be considered. If the patient does not have a deep overbite and if there is no need for torque control in either the anterior or posterior segments of the arches, the author recommends space closure mechanics using .019/.025 Nitinol archwires. These do not allow welding, so bracket attachments (hooks) are used for applying sliding mechanics.

A .008 ligature is used to lace the anterior teeth before engaging the archwire. This procedure prevents spaces opening in the anterior segment. First, the ligature is tied to the molars and then to an AlastiK™ module that has been slipped onto a hook on the canine

bracket, activating it by 3 mm (Fig. 4.42). This retraction system can remain in place for a maximum of 30 days, after which it should be replaced or activated. When the second molar is included in the treatment, tie the second molar to the first molar with metal ligatures.

Retraction with Nitinol springs

Space closure using sliding mechanics with a .019/.025 rectangular Nitinol archwire can also be carried out with Nitinol springs. It is very simple to assemble this system: one of the ends of the spring is first hooked onto the first molar, and then the other end is slipped onto the hook on the canine bracket (Fig. 4.43). To prevent anterior spaces from opening up, the clinician should place a .008 ligature wire from canine to canine before engaging the orthodontic archwire.

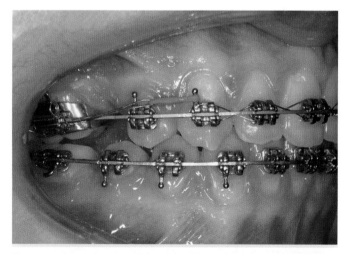

Fig. 4.42 Space closure applying sliding biomechanics using a .019/.025 Nitinol archwire. A laceback is placed from canine to canine underneath the archwire. The hook on the canine bracket is used to hold the AlastiK™ module.

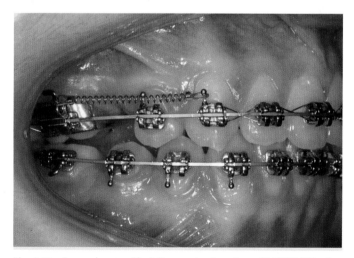

Fig. 4.43 Space closure with sliding mechanics using a .019/.025 Nitinol archwire and Nitinol spring.

Space closure mechanics using springs allows longer intervals between appointments. It also provides better control of the force applied, because there is a continuous force acting throughout the period of its application. When the second molar is included in the treatment, it is recommended to tie the second molar to the first molar using a metal ligature (Fig. 4.44).

Final stage of retraction

Once the residual spaces at the extraction sites have been closed, the retraction system should be left in place for an extra appointment. This procedure allows the roots to express the angulation built into the bracket. If this is not done, small spaces may open up in the extraction sites.

After leaving the retraction system in place for an extra appointment, a figure-of-eight metal ligature should be placed (passive laceback) from the hook welded on the mesial of the canine to the last tooth included in the appliance.[3] This procedure allows the torque to be transferred from the brackets to the roots without the need to apply any additional mechanics, such as Class II or Class III elastics, headgear, etc. This stage of treatment is called the **torque settling stage** (Figs 4.45 & 4.46).

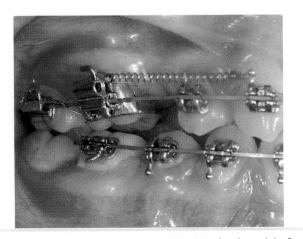

Fig. 4.44 Ligature placed between the upper second molar and the first molar when using the Nitinol spring retraction system.

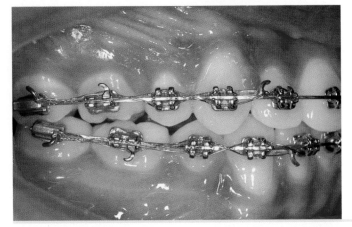
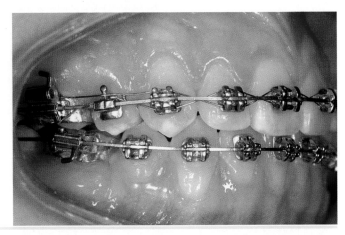

Figs 4.45 & 4.46 After space closure in the extraction sites, it is recommended to remove the retraction system and place passive ligatures to keep the spaces closed. When using a stainless steel archwire retraction system, place a laceback from the last tooth included in the appliance to the hook on the mesial of the canine on both sides. Fig. 4.46: When using a Nitinol archwire retraction system, place a ligature from molar to molar underneath the archwire.

Finishing and detailing

Before commencing settling of the occlusion, several aspects of the orthodontic treatment should be evaluated: the molar, premolar and canine interarch relationships; the midlines; root parallelism (using the panoramic X-ray); cephalometric measurements and the facial profile (using the cephalometric X-ray); contact points; curve of Spee; curve of Wilson;[11] canine and incisor overjet; alignment of the arches; functional aspects of the occlusion and the temporomandibular joints. After evaluating all these

aspects the final stage of treatment – finishing and detailing – can be initiated. Final settling of the occlusion should be done using .019/.025 braided rectangular archwires in both arches. The flexibility of the braided archwires allows minor vertical dental adjustments, which improves intercuspation of the teeth. However, before placing the braided archwires, the clinician should lace all teeth with a .008 metal ligature to prevent spaces from opening during the settling mechanics (Figs 4.47, 4.48 & 4.49). If the

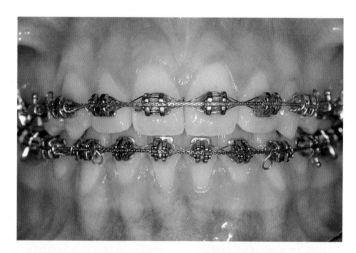

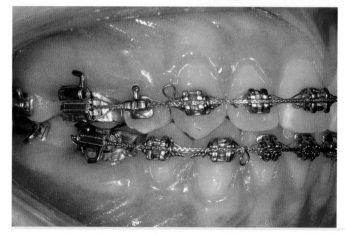
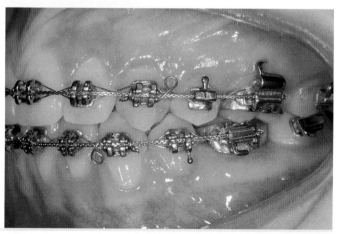

Figs 4.47, 4.48 & 4.49 Tying in the .008 metal ligature before inserting a .019/.025 rectangular braided archwire to start the settling stage. If the second molars are in good occlusion, they should be excluded from the set-up in the settling stage.

occlusion of the second molars is satisfactory, there is no need to include them in this stage of the treatment. Then the .019/.025 braided archwire should be inserted and the patient asked to wear 3/16 inch (4 ounce) elastics for 15 days followed by wearing of elastics at night only for another 15 days.

The SmartClip™ Self-Ligating Appliance features hooks on the distal wing of the canine and premolar brackets, which provides easy placement of the finishing elastics (Fig. 4.50).

After checking the functional goals of the occlusion in centric relation, protrusive functional movements by checking the incisor guidance, and lateroprotrusive functional movements by checking the canine guidance, the appliance can be removed (Figs 4.51, 4.52 & 4.53).

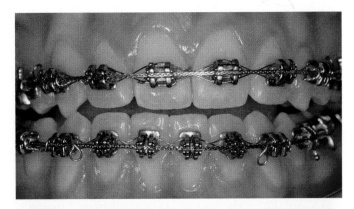

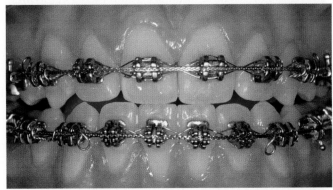

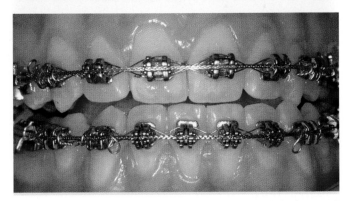

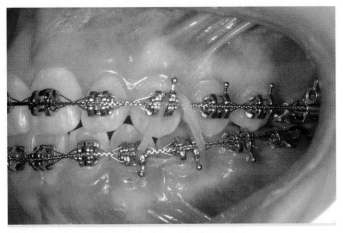

Fig. 4.50   Hooks on the distal wings of the SmartClip™ Self-Ligating brackets for easy placement of the finishing elastics.

Figs 4.51, 4.52 & 4.53   After settling of the occlusion, check the functional guidance – incisor guidance and canine guidance – and then remove the appliances.

Orthodontic retainers

The type of appliance used for retention is governed by patient comfort and the original malocclusion. When a lower 3–3 or 4–4 fixed retainer is to be used, first remove the upper appliance (Fig. 4.54). Then, after 30 days remove the lower appliance, and proceed with placement of the retainer previously selected for retention (Figs 4.55, 4.56 & 4.57) This protocol should be followed as there will be no retention for the lower posterior teeth, and it allows the masticatory activity and muscular action to influence the upper posterior teeth and adjust the lingual occlusion before removal of the lower appliance.

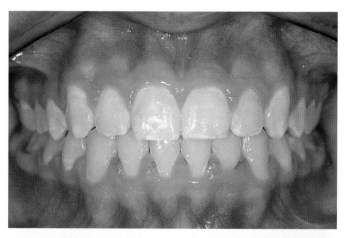

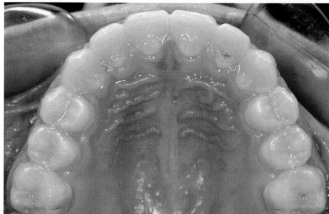

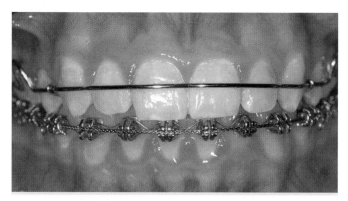

Fig. 4.54   The upper appliance should be removed first, and the lower appliance at the following appointment. This protocol is necessary because there will be no retention for the lower posterior teeth. The upper removable retainer should be placed immediately after the removal of the appliance from the upper arch.

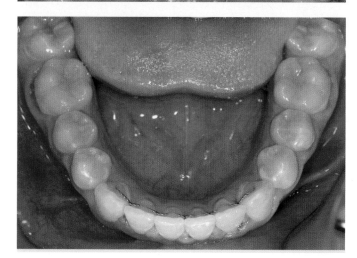

Figs 4.55, 4.56 & 4.57   Frontal and occlusal views of the upper arch and occlusal view of the lower arch with 3–3 fixed retainer on the lower arch after appliance removal.

Upper arch

Removable acrylic retainers are used for upper arch retention, and can be used along with individual bonded retainers to prevent relapse of rotations or a diastema. The retainer, a modified Hawley wraparound retainer, is made with a continuous buccal wire that goes all the way around the last erupted tooth (distal of the first or second molars) on each side (Fig. 4.58). Functional movements should be possible without the lower teeth coming into contact with the retainer when the patient closes the mouth in maximal intercuspation (Figs 4.59, 4.60 & 4.61).

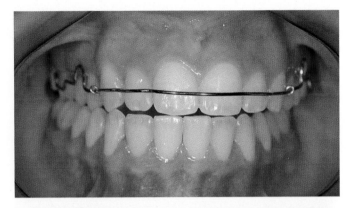

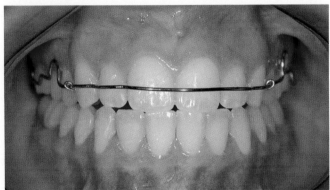

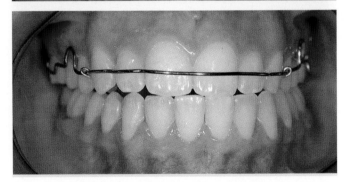

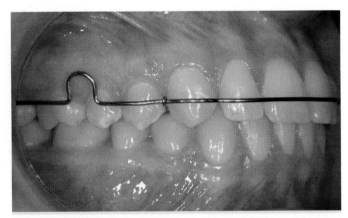

Fig. 4.58 A modified Hawley retainer with continuous buccal wire going all the way around the last erupted tooth on each side.

Figs 4.59, 4.60 & 4.61 The upper removable retainer should allow the execution of the functional movements. The lower teeth should not come into contact with the retainer in maximal intercuspation.

Fixed retainers can be used in the upper arch for patients with periodontal problems or with a persistent diastema. Such retainers can be used along with the removable upper retainers (Figs 4.62 & 4.63).

Lower arch

Retention of the lower arch requires good planning and depends on the orthodontic treatment mechanics applied, the comfort of the patient and the original malocclusion.

There are two types of retainer for the lower arch: fixed and removable. The use of fixed retainers is recommended for cases in which the lower arch did not require expansion during treatment. If expansion was required, removable retainers should be used. If there were no premolar extractions, canine to canine retainers made of .016 twist-flex wire should be used (Fig. 4.64). When stiffer retention is required, retainers can be made with .018 stainless steel wire, with relief at the contact points. This type of retainer[12] is comfortable for the patient, and allows good hygiene and the use of dental floss (Fig. 4.65). For patients with

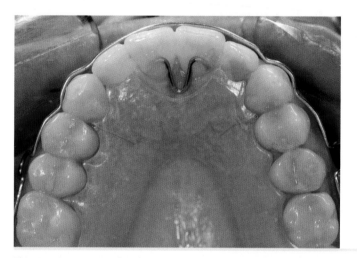

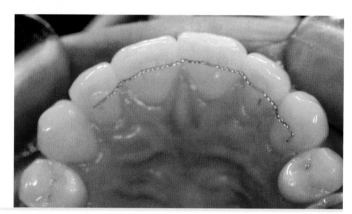

Figs 4.62 & 4.63   Fixed retainers in the upper arch. These can be used along with a removable retainer.

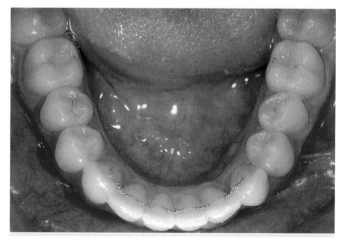

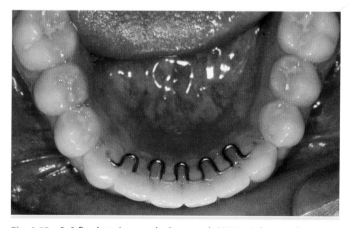

Fig. 4.64   Occlusal view of 3–3 fixed retainer on the lower arch (.016 twist-flex archwire) in a non-extraction case.

Fig. 4.65   3–3 fixed retainer on the lower arch (.018 stainless steel archwire) with relief at the contact points. This retainer is more hygienic and comfortable for the patient.

periodontal problems (i.e. gingival inflammation), canine to canine removable retainers are preferred (Fig. 4.66). For premolar extraction cases, retainers from canine to canine, or from second premolar to second premolar bonded on the mesial fossae of the teeth can be used (Figs 4.67 & 4.68).

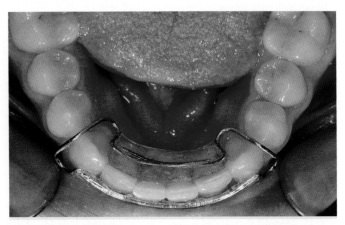

Fig. 4.66   3–3 removable retainer with a resin shield provides better hygiene and comfort for the patient.

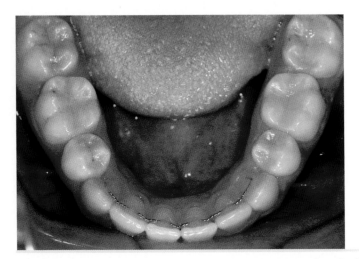

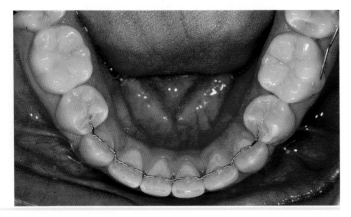

Figs 4.67 & 4.68   3–3 fixed retainer in premolar extraction cases and 4–4 fixed retainer in a premolar extraction case.

References

1. Andrews L F 1989 Straight-Wire: the concept and appliance. L A Wells, San Diego, p 407

2. Roth R H 1996 Mecânica do tratamento para aparelho straight-wire. In: Graber T M, Vanarsdall R L Jr (eds) Ortodontia: princípios e técnicas atuais, 2nd edn. Guanabara Koogan, Rio de Janeiro, pp 636–660

3. McLaughlin R P, Bennett J C, Trevisi H J 2001 Systemized orthodontic treatment mechanics. Mosby, Edinburgh

4. Sebata E 1980 An orthodontic study of teeth and dental arch form on the Japanese normal occlusion. Shikwa Gakuho 80:945–969

5. Watanabe K, Koga M, Yatabe K, Motegi E, Isshiki Y A 1996 A morphometric study on setup models of Japanese malocclusions. Shikwa Gakuho 96:209–222

6. Bennett J C, McLaughlin R P 1990 Controlled space closure with a preadjusted appliance system. Journal of Clinical Orthodontics 10:251–260

7. Trevisi H J 2005 The SmartClip™ self-ligating appliance system. Technique Guide. 3M Company

8. Zanelato R 1993 Evaluation of the loss of anchorage of the lower first molar in cases treated with extractions of the first and second premolars with the Straight Wire technique. Revista Straight Wire Brasil III: 12–21.

9. von Spee F G 1890 The condylar path of the mandible in the glenoid fossa. Kiel, Germany

10. Moresca R, Vigorito J W 2005 Avaliação in vitro da degradação da força produzida por módulos elásticos utilizados no fechamento de espaço com a mecânica por deslizamento. Ortodontia Soc Paulista Ortodontia 38:212–218

11. Wilson G H 1911 Manual of dental prosthetics. Lea and Febiger, Philadelphia

12. Bicalho J S 2002 Description of fixed retention with free access to the use of dental floss. Revista Dental Press de Ortodontia e Ortopedia Facial 1:9–13

CHAPTER 4 CLINICAL CASE

Name: LO
Sex: Female
Age: 15.1 years
Facial pattern: Dolichofacial
Skeletal pattern: Class I

Diagnosis

A 2 mm Class II molar relationship on the right side, Class I molar relation on the left side, upper midline deviation to the right side, buccally erupted upper right canine with arch discrepancy and crowding in the lower arch.

Treatment plan

Extraction of the lower right and left first premolars and upper left first premolar with appropriate treatment mechanics aimed at correcting the upper midline deviation and relieving the lower crowding. Following upper midline correction, extraction of the upper right first premolar and use of additional mechanics to achieve a Class I molar relationship on both sides.

Appliance

- Upper palatal bar
- Lower lingual arch
- SmartClip™ Self-Ligating Appliance
- Upper modified Hawley wraparound retainer
- Lower 3–3 fixed retainer

Case report

The patient presented with a 2 mm Class II molar relationship on the right side and a Class I molar relationship on the left side, severe lower crowding, buccally erupted upper right canine and upper midline deviation to the right side.

The initial treatment plan consisted of extraction of both the lower first premolars and the upper left first premolar with the aim of relieving the lower crowding and correcting the upper midline. An upper palatal bar and lower lingual arch were used for anchorage and the SmartClip™ Self-Ligating Appliance was partially set up in both arches before carrying out the extractions.

In the aligning stage, .014 and .016 classic Nitinol archwires were used. Sliding mechanics with active lacebacks were used until the alignment of the lower arch was finalized and the upper midline was corrected. Then the upper right first premolar was extracted, and the upper arch aligned using a .016 classic Nitinol archwire.

After finalizing alignment on the upper right side, the lingual arch was removed but the palatal bar was kept in place. Buccal tubes were bonded on the upper and lower second molars and .019/.025 Nitinol archwires used for leveling.

Space closure was carried out with sliding mechanics on a .019/.025 stainless steel archwire with hooks welded mesial to the canines. The retraction system used consisted of AlastiK™ modules tied to metal ligatures. For final detailing, the palatal bar was removed and some brackets repositioned. After re-leveling, the remaining spaces were closed using rectangular archwires.

The occlusion was settled with .019/.025 braided archwires in both arches after removing the buccal tubes from the second molars. Vertical finishing elastics were used for 21 days, 24 hours per day and then at night only for another 21 days. A removable retainer was placed in the upper arch and a 3–3 retainer in the lower arch. Good vertical positioning and good torque were achieved in the lower incisors.

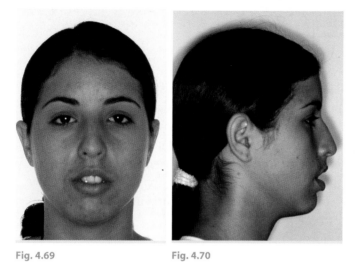

Fig. 4.69   Fig. 4.70

Figs 4.69 & 4.70
Pretreatment photographs showing facial symmetry,
Class I facial profile and lack of lip seal.

Figs 4.71, 4.72 & 4.73
Cephalometric X-ray, measurements and tracing
showing increased vertical height and therefore
increased ANB.

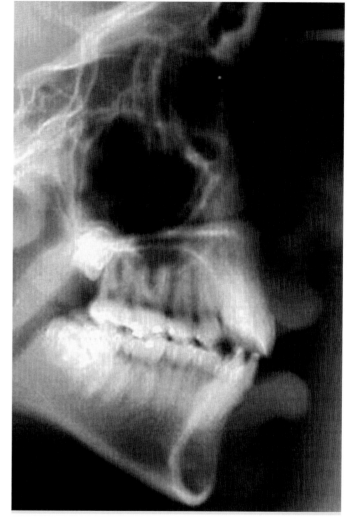

Fig. 4.71

Figs 4.74, 4.75 & 4.76
Pretreatment intraoral photographs showing a mild
Class II molar relationship on the right side, a Class I
molar relationship on the left side and upper midline
deviation to the right side.

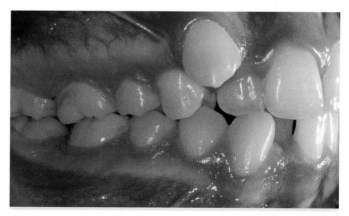

Fig. 4.74

SNA ∠	73°
SNB ∠	68°
ANB ∠	5°
A-N ⊥ FH	1 mm
Po-N ⊥ FH	–10 mm
Wits	2 mm
GoGn SN ∠	46°
FH Md ∠	31°
Mx Md ∠	34°
U1 to A-Po	7 mm
L1 to A-Po	4 mm
U1 to Mx plane ∠	105°
L1 to Md plane ∠	94°

Facial analysis

Nasolabial ∠	95°
NA ⊥ nose	30 mm
Lip thickness	13 mm

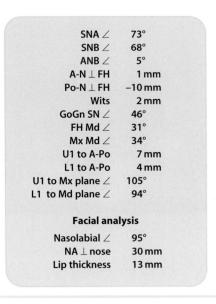

Fig. 4.72

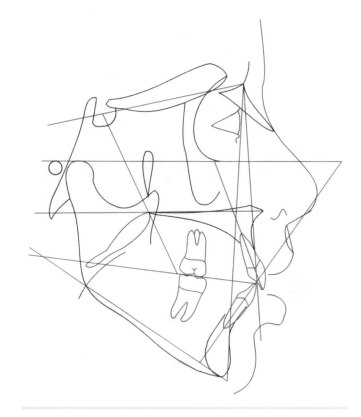

Fig. 4.73

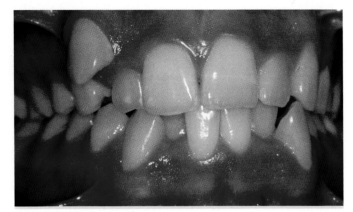

Fig. 4.75

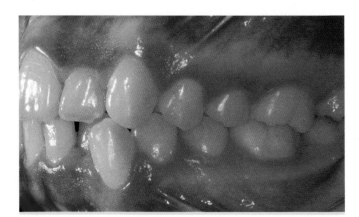

Fig. 4.76

Figs 4.77, 4.78
Pretreatment upper and lower occlusal views showing buccal eruption of the upper right canine and severe lower crowding.

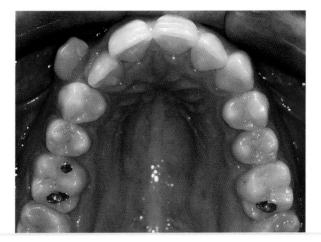

Fig. 4.77

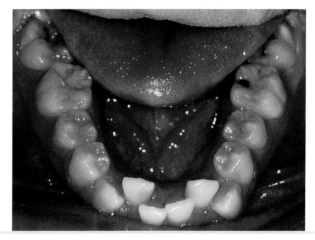

Fig. 4.78

Figs 4.80, 4.81, 4.82, 4.83 & 4.84
Upper midline correction started with active lacebacks. An open coil spring placed between the upper right incisor and the first premolar to correct the midline deviation. SmartClip™ Self-Ligating Appliance with palatal bar and lingual arch. A .014 round Nitinol archwire is in place to begin alignment.

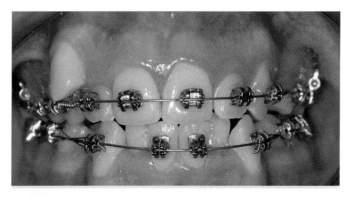

Fig. 4.80

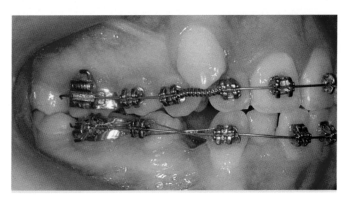

Fig. 4.81

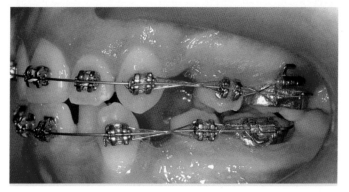

Fig. 4.82

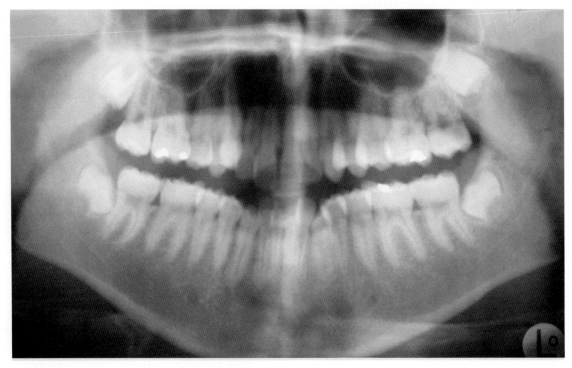

Fig. 4.79

Fig. 4.79
Panoramic X-ray showing full permanent dentition with lack of space for the developing lower third molars.

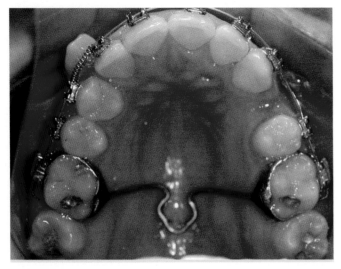

Fig. 4.83

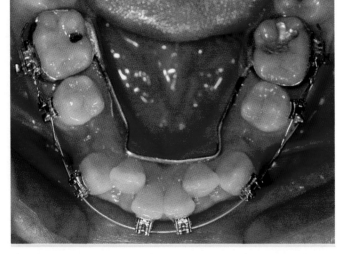

Fig. 4.84

Figs 4.85, 4.86 & 4.87
Lower lateral incisors bonded with .016 round Nitinol superelastic archwire. Aligning mechanics and upper midline correction continued.

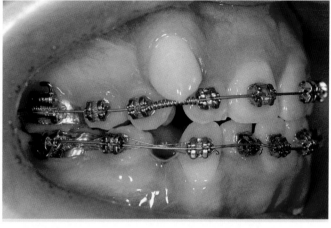

Fig. 4.85

Figs 4.88 & 4.89
Upper and lower occlusal views of .016 rounded Nitinol archwire, bonded lower lateral incisors and continuing aligning mechanics. Palatal bar and lingual arch in place to maintain the anchorage.

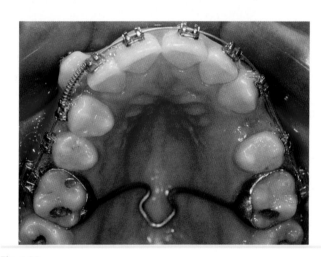

Fig. 4.88

Figs 4.90, 4.91 & 4.92
Finishing the first aligning stage with .016 Nitinol archwire. The upper midline has been corrected and the canines have been distalized to align the incisors.

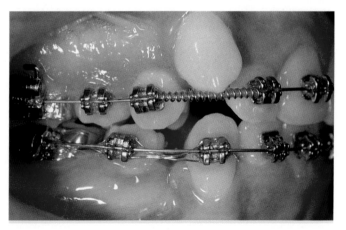

Fig. 4.90

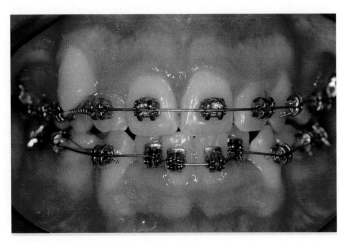

Fig. 4.86

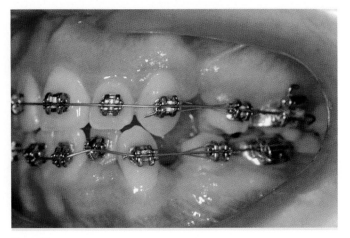

Fig. 4.87

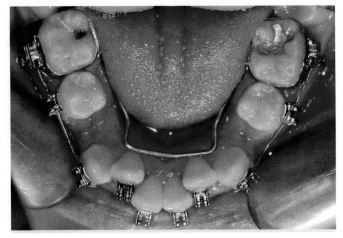

Fig. 4.89

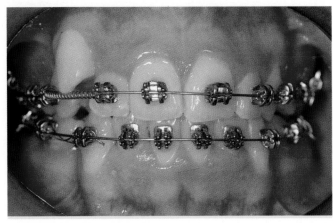

Fig. 4.91

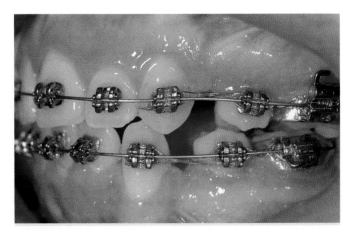

Fig. 4.92

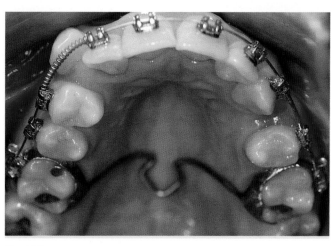

Fig. 4.93

Figs 4.93 & 4.94
Upper and lower occlusal views of the end of the first aligning stage.

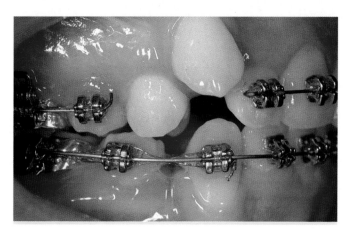

Fig. 4.95

Figs 4.95, 4.96 & 4.97
Upper and lower arches before the extraction of the upper right first premolar. The lower archwire was kept in place and the upper archwire was segmented to maintain the alignment of the upper bracket slots.

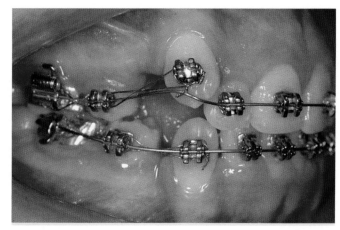

Fig. 4.98

Figs 4.98, 4.99 & 4.100
After the extraction of the upper right first premolar, a .014 Nitinol archwire was engaged and lacebacks used to align the upper right canine.

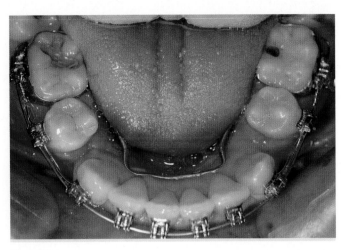

Fig. 4.94

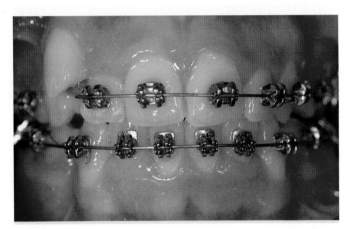

Fig. 4.96

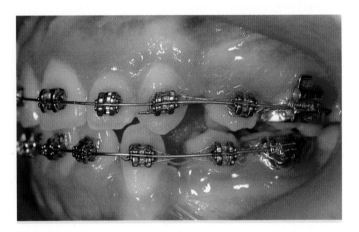

Fig. 4.97

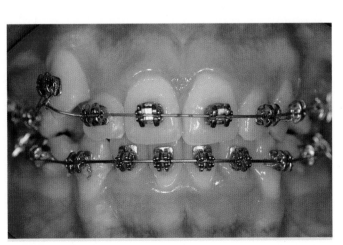

Fig. 4.99

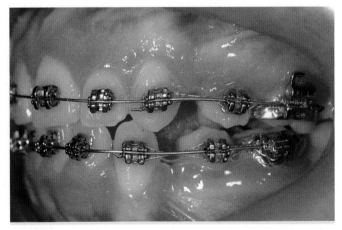

Fig. 4.100

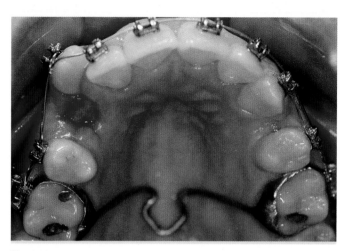

Figs 4.101 & 4.102
Upper and lower occlusal views showing the mechanics for alignment of the upper right canine. A .016 Nitinol archwire is present in the lower arch with passive lacebacks. Note the distalization of the lower canines to align the incisors and maintenance of anchorage. The lingual arch has been removed.

Fig. 4.101

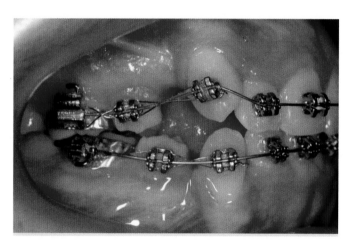

Figs 4.103, 4.104 & 4.105
Intermediate phase of the second aligning stage. The upper archwire is in the bracket slot of the upper right canine.

Fig. 4.103

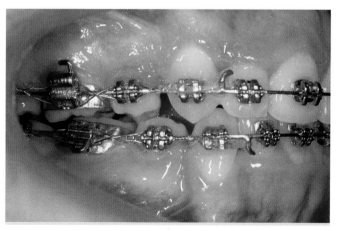

Figs 4.106, 4.107 & 4.108
Space closure with .019/.025 rectangular stainless steel archwire and hooks welded mesial to the canines. The retraction system consisted of metal ligatures tied to AlastiK™ modules.

Fig. 4.106

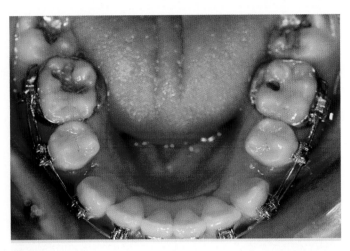

Fig. 4.102

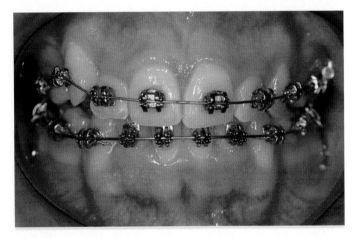

Fig. 4.104

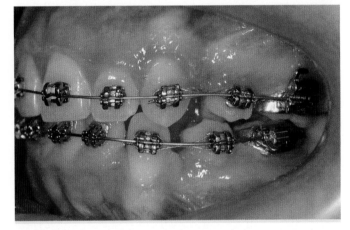

Fig. 4.105

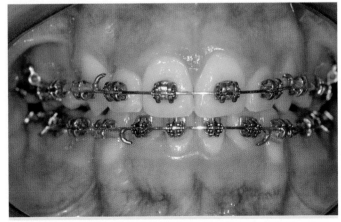

Fig. 4.107

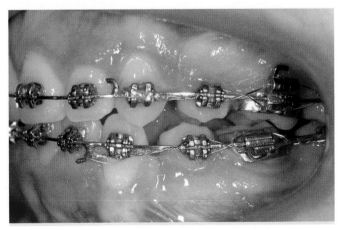

Fig. 4.108

Figs 4.109 & 4.110
Upper and lower occlusal views showing .019/.025 rectangular stainless steel archwires and use of sliding mechanics to close the remaining spaces.

Figs 4.111, 4.112 & 4.113
Finalizing space closure. There are passive lacebacks in the lower arch to maintain the space closure in the extraction sites.

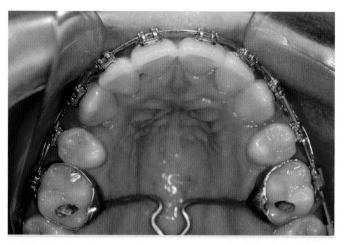

Fig. 4.109

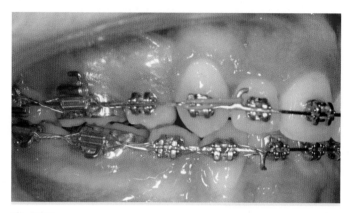

Fig. 4.111

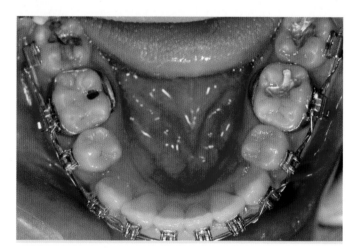

Fig. 4.110

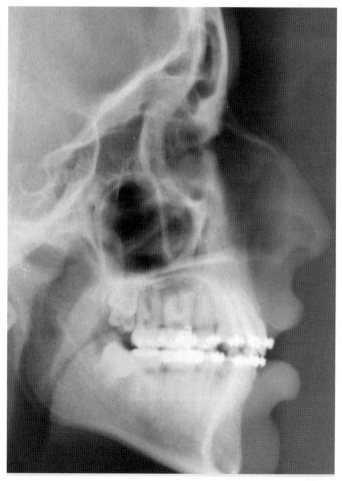

Figs 4.114, 4.115 & 4.116
Interim cephalometric X-ray, tracing and measurements showing good vertical control and good torque control of the lower incisors.

Fig. 4.114

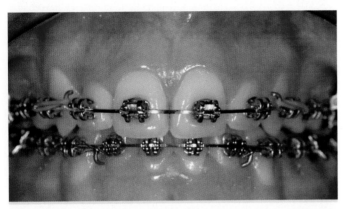

Fig. 4.112

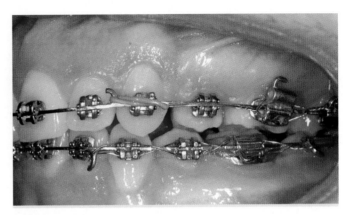

Fig. 4.113

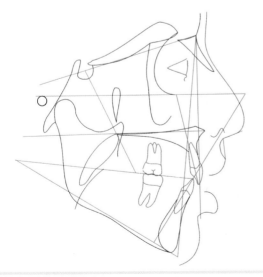

Fig. 4.115

Fig. 4.116

SNA ∠	73°
SNB ∠	68°
ANB ∠	5°
A-N ⊥ FH	1 mm
Po-N ⊥ FH	−10 mm
Wits	5 mm
GoGn SN ∠	46°
FH Md ∠	31°
Mx Md ∠	32°
U1 to A-Po	6 mm
L1 to A-Po	2 mm
U1 to Mx plane ∠	103°
L1 to Md plane ∠	92°

Facial analysis

Nasolabial ∠	104°
NA ⊥ nose	28 mm
Lip thickness	14 mm

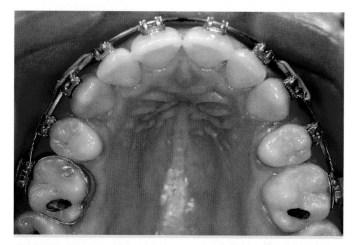

Fig. 4.117

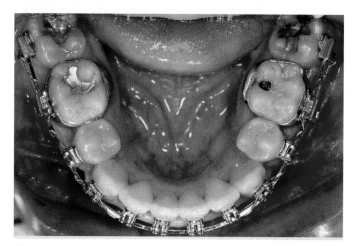

Fig. 4.118

Figs 4.117 & 4.118
Upper and lower occlusal views after closure of spaces in the extraction sites. Note the good arch form, alignment and contact points.

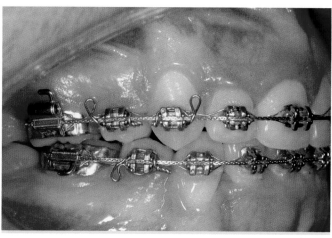

Fig. 4.120

Figs 4.120, 4.121 & 4.122
Settling the occlusion with .019/.025 braided archwire. The upper and lower second molar tubes have been removed.

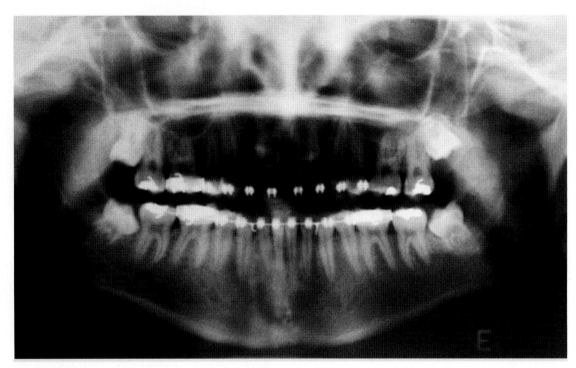

Fig. 4.119

Fig. 4.119
Panoramic X-ray shows the positioning of the roots.

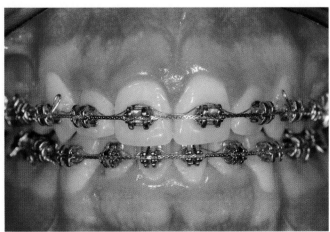

Fig. 4.121

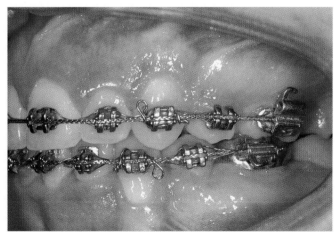

Fig. 4.122

Figs 4.123 & 4.124
Upper and lower occlusal views during the final stage of treatment. The second molar buccal tubes have been removed.

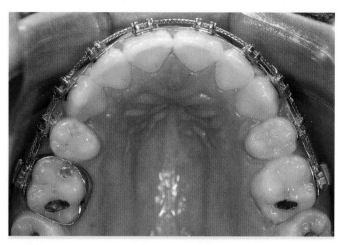

Fig. 4.123

Figs 4.125, 4.126 & 4.127
Post-treatment intraoral photographs showing good finishing, Class I molar and canine relationships on the right and left side, and upper midline correction.

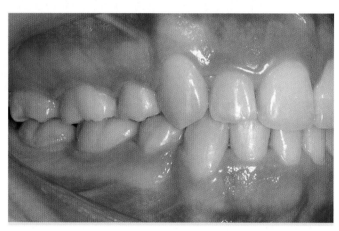

Fig. 4.125

Figs 4.128, 4.129 & 4.130
Upper and lower post-treatment occlusal views and frontal view showing good arch form, alignment, and contact points, a modified wraparound Hawley-type retainer in the upper arch and a 3–3 fixed retainer in the lower arch. Figure 4.130 shows the anterior guidance and the cuspid guidance achieved at the orthodontic treatment.

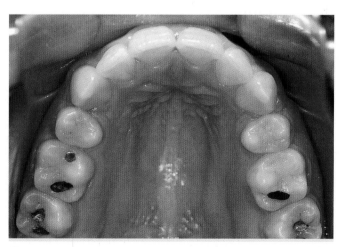

Fig. 4.128

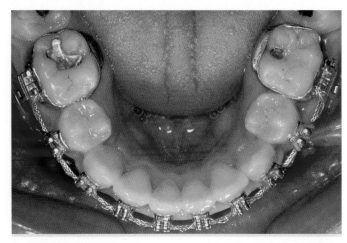

Fig. 4.124

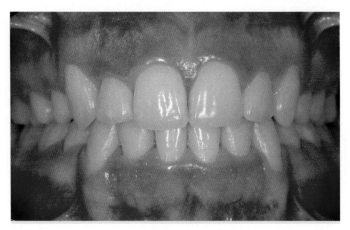

Fig. 4.126

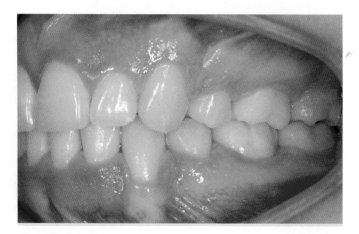

Fig. 4.127

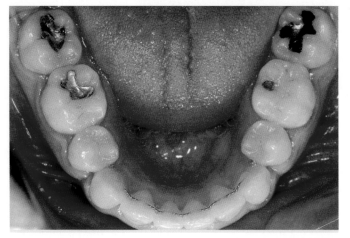

Fig. 4.129

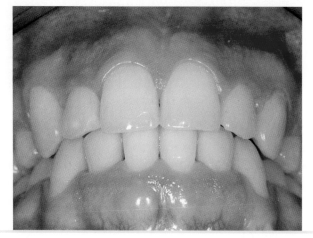

Fig. 4.130

Figs 4.131 & 4.132
Post-treatment frontal and profile photographs
showing facial symmetry and good lip seal.

Figs 4.133 & 4.134
Post-treatment three-quarter views with and without
smile showing a good facial and smile line balance.

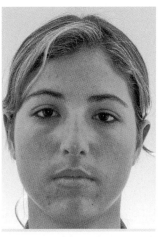

Fig. 4.131

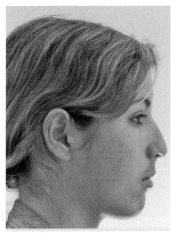

Fig. 4.132

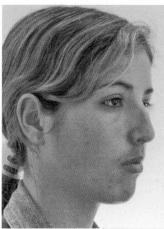

Fig. 4.133

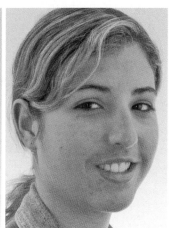

Fig. 4.134

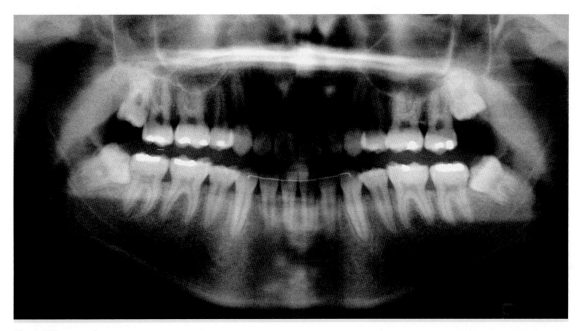

Fig. 4.135

Fig. 4.135
Post-treatment panoramic X-ray showing the position
of the roots and impacted third molars.

Figs 4.136, 4.137, 4.138 & 4.139
Post-treatment cephalometric X-ray, tracing and
cephalometric measurements showing a good
orthodontic treatment result. Superimposition of the
initial and final cephalometric tracings on SN shows
good vertical control and well-positioned lower
incisors.

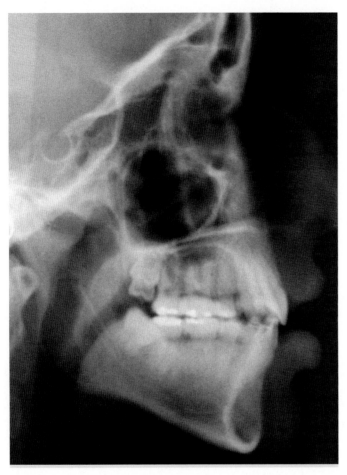

Fig. 4.136

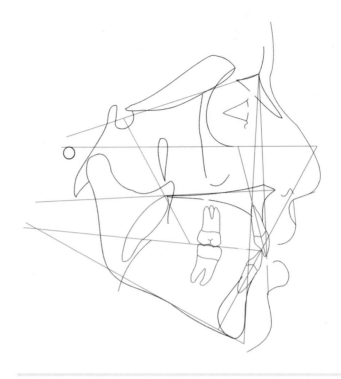

Fig. 4.137

SNA ∠	73°	
SNB ∠	69°	
ANB ∠	4°	
A-N ⊥ FH	2 mm	
Po-N ⊥ FH	−7 mm	
Wits	3.5 mm	
GoGn SN ∠	44°	
FH Md ∠	28°	
Mx Md ∠	31°	
U1 to A-Po	5 mm	
L1 to A-Po	2 mm	
U1 to Mx plane ∠	102°	
L1 to Md plane ∠	91°	

Facial analysis

Nasolabial ∠	103°
NA ⊥ nose	29 mm
Lip thickness	13 mm

Fig. 4.138

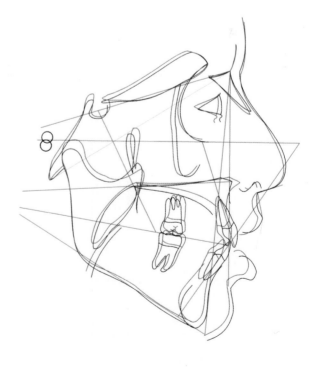

Fig. 4.139

Versatility of the SmartClip™ Self-Ligating Appliance

Versatility

In orthodontics, versatility describes an orthodontic technique that allows changing the positioning of a tooth or a group of teeth – angulation, rotation and torque – without investing in additional brackets.

The developers of the MBT™ Appliance System, McLaughlin, Bennett and Trevisi, included versatility in the MBT™ technique, with the aim of having a single orthodontic bracket prescription for several types of malocclusion as well as for individual overcorrections.[1]

Thus, versatility of an orthodontic technique allows customization of tooth positioning, with the aim of overcorrecting the malocclusion. A single bracket can be positioned in different ways on the same tooth, or brackets and buccal tubes meant for one tooth type can be used on another tooth type. Versatility also minimizes the need for first, second and third order bends in the archwires during all stages of treatment. Horizontal positioning (in–out) and rotation, angulation and inclination (torque), which represent the first, second and third order bends, respectively, added to the archwire in the Edgewise technique, are already incorporated into the brackets of preadjusted appliances.[1,2] However, it is important to recognize that, despite using a versatile technique, certain cases will require customization of treatment. For instance, in cases with variations in the shape of the crowns, additional bends may be needed to compensate for the abnormal shape. Third order bends (additional torque) may be needed depending on the severity of the malocclusion and the treatment mechanics applied.

The SmartClip™ Self-Ligating Appliance[3] has the same tip and torque specifications as the MBT™ Appliance System[1] and therefore the same versatility. This versatility can be applied during the initial or final stages of orthodontic treatment when using the SmartClip™ Self-Ligating Appliance.

It is important to understand that an orthodontic technique is considered **versatile** when it does not have rotational control in the prescription of the brackets, so allowing rotational overcorrection.

180° bracket rotation in cases with crossbite of the upper lateral incisor, providing –10° torque

It is common to have patients with lingually displaced lateral incisors. The cause is usually lack of space in the upper arch or excessive tooth size (Bolton discrepancy[4]) in the upper anterior segment, which often occur in Class I or Class III malocclusions.

In 1911, Lischer[5] suggested a method of classifying individual tooth malpositions. He used the suffix 'version' to define the direction of deviation of a tooth's position in relation to its normal position. Accordingly, linguoversion is the term used to describe a tooth's position when it is positioned lingual to its normal position.

In the normal mixed dentition, the permanent lateral incisors develop lingual to the central incisors after the centrals have reached the occlusal plane. Therefore, these teeth begin erupting from their most lingual position in relation to the centrals. When the upper lateral incisors reach the occlusal plane, it marks the end of the first transitional period, as defined by van der Linden.[6] Thus, when there is lack of space in the anterior region of the maxilla for the eruption of the permanent teeth, the lateral incisors erupt in linguoversion, because they develop behind the centrals and erupt later (Figs 5.1, 5.2 & 5.3).

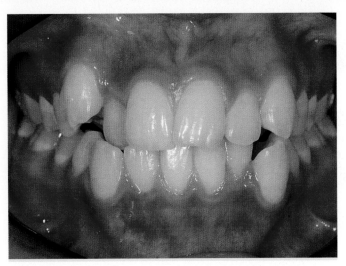

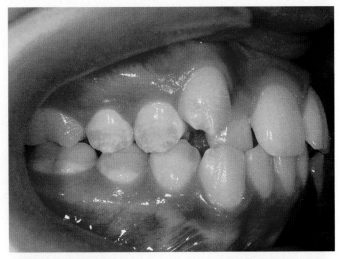

Figs 5.1, 5.2 & 5.3 A Class I malocclusion with lack of space for the anterior teeth and crossbite of the upper right lateral incisor (lingually displaced incisor).

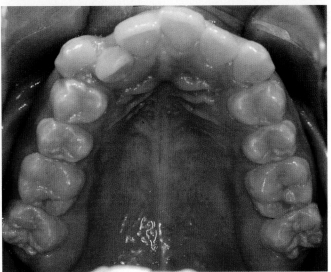

Space management

As linguoversion of the upper lateral incisors is related to a lack of space in the upper arch, precise treatment planning and mechanics are necessary to produce sufficient space. Space can be gained by expansion, by moving the incisors labially, by enamel stripping or by extractions. The best choice in each case will be different and will depend on the crowding and the patient's facial pattern.

Patients showing horizontal facial growth can often benefit from an increase in arch length, thus avoiding the need for extraction of premolars. The anterior region of the jaws, especially the mandibular symphysis, is larger in brachyfacial individuals and often allows extensive movement of the incisor teeth. In this facial pattern, the upper and lower incisors will be more labially inclined at the end of treatment due to the counterclockwise rotation of the mandible.[7] Treatment for these patients is generally customized and often requires a non-extraction approach. Open coil springs are used to create the necessary space.[1] The spring is placed during aligning and leveling, when an .016 or .018 Nitinol or stainless steel

archwire is used. It is also recommended to place metal ligatures on the brackets adjacent to the spring to avoid inadvertent tooth rotations. The distal bends on the leveling archwires should not be tight, otherwise they will restrict the labial movement of the incisor teeth. So leave a small gap between the molar tube and the distal bend to provide some freedom of movement for an increase in dental arch length (Figs 5.4 & 5.5).

Extractions, especially premolar extractions, are another way of making space. Patients with vertical facial growth pattern and minor open bite, or those showing good growth pattern and crowding greater

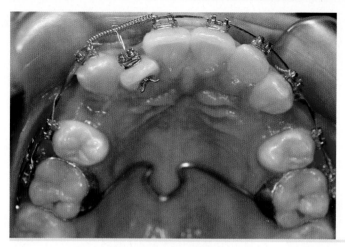
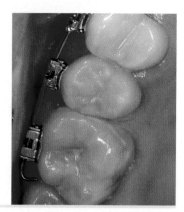

Figs 5.4 & 5.5   SmartClip™ Self-Ligating Appliance with the lateral incisor bracket rotated 180°, open coil spring and distal bend, with a gap distal to the molar tube.

than or equal to 7 mm can benefit from premolar extractions. Individual retraction of the canines into the extraction site is often recommended to create the necessary space to correct crowding of lateral incisors. There are several methods of retracting canines, such as with Nitinol springs or elastic chains. Customized lacebacks[8] (Fig. 5.6) on the canines is an often applied method. For these lacebacks, .009 (.23 mm) ligatures are used, and they should be placed at the beginning of the aligning stage.[1] The lacebacks move the crown distally and the archwire uprights the root. Open coil springs can be used along with lacebacks to open anterior spaces.[1]

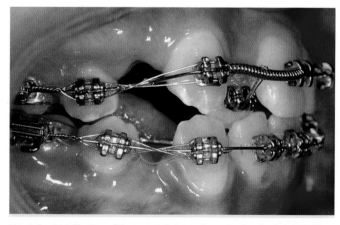

Fig. 5.6   Distalization of the upper right canine using lacebacks, to create space for the lingually positioned upper right lateral incisor.

Bracket specification

The introduction of the preadjusted Straight-Wire™ appliance by Andrews[9] at the beginning of the 1970s represented a milestone in modern orthodontics. Andrews' research on normal natural occlusions also found some common and reliable characteristics among normal occlusions that could be consistently reproduced by use of preadjusted orthodontic appliances when treating malocclusions. One of these 'six keys' to a normal occlusion is the inclination of dental crowns. Crown inclination is the angle formed by a line perpendicular to the occlusal plane and the tangent to the center of the buccal (or labial) surface of the clinical crown. It varies in value as positive and negative depending on the group of teeth being considered. Thus, the inclination of the crowns of the upper anterior teeth is positive, because the incisal portion of the crown is located towards the labial in relation to the cervical, whereas it is negative from canines through to molars. In the upper arch, the lingual inclination is steady and similar from canines to second premolars and slightly more pronounced in the molars. In the lower arch, the lingual inclination increases progressively from canines to second molars.

Among the 120 models with normal occlusion used by Andrews during the development of the preadjusted appliance, for the upper lateral incisors, the average inclination of the crowns was 4.42° (maximum 17° and minimum −6°). The average angulation of the clinical crowns was 8.04° (maximum 15° and minimum −2°). On analyzing this data, it becomes evident that there is great variability in the measurements. Although the preadjusted appliance is recommended for use in all cases, in some situations it is necessary to incorporate bends in the archwires to compensate for or overcorrect tooth positions.

In 2003, Trevisi Zanelato[10] conducted a study to evaluate the values of the angulation and inclination of tooth crowns in the Brazilian population, with the aim of comparing these values with Andrews' values. The sample comprised 60 individuals from 12 to 21 years of age. These individuals had normal natural occlusion (without prior orthodontic intervention). The measurements of the crowns of the upper lateral incisors were as follows: average inclination 4.48° (maximum 17° and minimum −5°); average angulation 6.19° (maximum 19° and minimum −2°). These values are close to those found by Andrews.

Figure 5.7 shows angulation and torque (inclination) recommended for the upper lateral incisors. Angulations of several bracket prescriptions available on the market are shown, presenting a variability of 1°. In contrast, there is wide variation in the

recommended torque, which shows a variability of 11° between the 3° suggested by Andrews and the 14° recommended by Ricketts.[11] The reason for such great variability in the torque recommendations is because the original Straight-Wire™ Appliance is essentially based on the final positions of teeth found in normal natural occlusions. In the other prescriptions, additional torque was added to the brackets of anterior teeth to compensate for the torque loss often seen during treatment, for example, in treatment of Class II malocclusions.

The SmartClip™ Self-Ligating Appliance prescription features numerous modifications compared with the original Straight-Wire™ Appliance. The angulation of the dental crowns is reduced by 1° to minimize the increase in arch length that could occur during the initial stages of treatment with a preadjusted appliance. The additional torque compensates for torque loss that frequently occurs in some treatments. Thus, for the lateral incisors, 8° of angulation and 10° of inclination are recommended, which is the same as the MBT™ prescription, but represents 7° of additional inclination compared with the original Straight-Wire™ Appliance.[1]

When applying the versatility of the SmartClip™ Self-Ligated Appliance to palatally displaced upper lateral incisors, a normal bracket should be rotated 180° before bonding.[1] As a result, the angulation is maintained but the crown inclination is changed, from +10° to −10° (Figs 5.8, 5.9 & 5.10). The goal of this maneuver is to move the palatally displaced root labially, placing it in a more stable position, thus avoiding relapse. It is important to recognize that the rotation of the lateral incisor bracket helps to reduce, but does not eliminate, the need to introduce third order bends in the rectangular archwires in all cases. Thus, during finishing and detailing, the clinician should carefully observe the crown inclination of the upper lateral incisor and then decide whether compensatory third order bends are required in the final archwires.

Upper lateral incisor	Tip	Torque
Ricketts	8°	14°
Andrews	9°	3°
Roth	9°	8°
Alexander	8°	7°
MBT™	8°	10°
SmartClip™	8°	10°

Fig. 5.7 Angulation and torque values of various prescriptions for the upper lateral incisors.

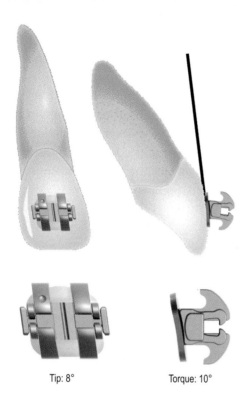

Fig. 5.8

Tip: 8°

Torque: 10°

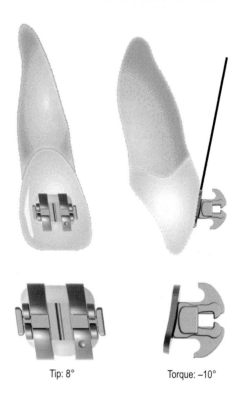

Tip: 8°

Torque: −10°

Fig. 5.9

Figs 5.8, 5.9 & 5.10 SmartClip™ Self-Ligating Appliance bracket specification for upper lateral incisors. Figure 5.8 shows the normal recommended bracket positioning. Figure 5.9 shows a bracket positioned after rotating 180° (appliance versatility). Figure 5.10 shows a bracket positioned after rotating 180° on a lateral incisor in the clinical situation.

Three torque options for the upper canines (−7°, 0°, +7°), and three torque options for the lower canines (−6°, 0°, +6°)

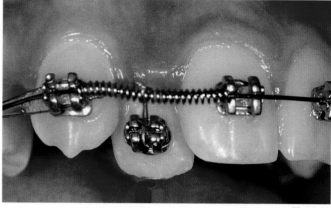

Fig. 5.10

One of the greatest challenges in orthodontics, as a specialty, is the relationship between esthetics and function, because, besides deciding on the best esthetics for a patient, clinicians also have the responsibility of providing a stable and functional occlusion for the patient.

The protective role of the canines in the lateroprotrusive movements of the mandible forms the basis of the concept of mutually protected occlusion.

These teeth are responsible for the protection of the posterior teeth during the lateral movements of the mandible, as they take the brunt of the horizontal forces, which can otherwise lead to long-term pathological changes. Thus, it is important that the canine crowns are well positioned both vertically and horizontally at the end of orthodontic treatment, so that they can perform their protective function efficiently. The recommended inclination for the canines is adequate for most cases. However, these values can be influenced by some variables such as arch shape, the morphology of the buccal surface, the vertical position of the bracket on the buccal surface and the canine position. Hence, it is the clinician's responsibility to identify these individual variables and add bends that may be needed to correctly position these teeth. It is necessary to customize the treatment according to the patient's facial characteristics and malocclusion.

Recommendations for canine crown inclination when using the SmartClip™ Self-Ligating Appliance

After several years of clinical experience with the preadjusted appliance, McLaughlin, Bennett and Trevisi[1] idealized the MBT™ Appliance System, introducing a range of improvements and specification changes to overcome the clinical shortcomings presented by the Straight-Wire™ prescription.[2] The

authors noted that the measurements of the 120 non-orthodontic normal cases evaluated by Andrews were of adult patients without extractions, but typical orthodontic cases are very different.

The inclination of −7° for the upper canines is considered satisfactory for most cases; however, the inclination of −11° in the original Straight-Wire™ Appliance for lower canines was not found to be appropriate. It showed a tendency to leave the roots of the lower canines buccally tipped in almost all cases. As a result, McLaughlin, Bennett and Trevisi developed two new brackets for the upper and lower canines with three torque options – positive inclination, zero degree, and negative inclination – providing nine combinations of inclination for the canines.[1] Such versatility helps to achieve the correct overjet for these teeth. Figures 5.11, 5.12, 5.13, 5.14, 5.15 & 5.16 show torque options for the upper and lower canines. To decide on the best option, there are some guidelines that should be followed:

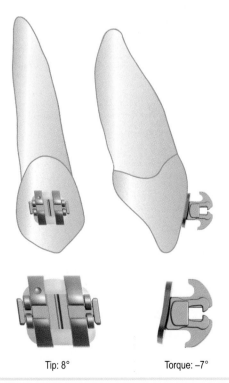

Tip: 8°   Torque: −7°

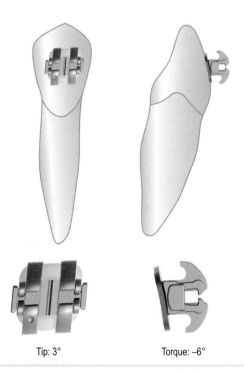

Tip: 3°   Torque: −6°

Figs 5.11 & 5.12   An upper canine bracket with 8° angulation and −7° torque and a lower canine bracket with 3° angulation and −6° torque positioned on the buccal surface of the respective tooth.

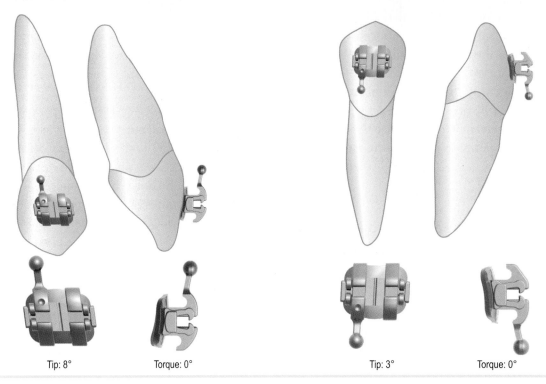

Tip: 8°   Torque: 0°   Tip: 3°   Torque: 0°

Figs 5.13 & 5.14   An upper canine bracket with 8° angulation and 0° torque and a lower canine bracket with 3° angulation and 0° torque positioned on the buccal surface of the respective tooth.

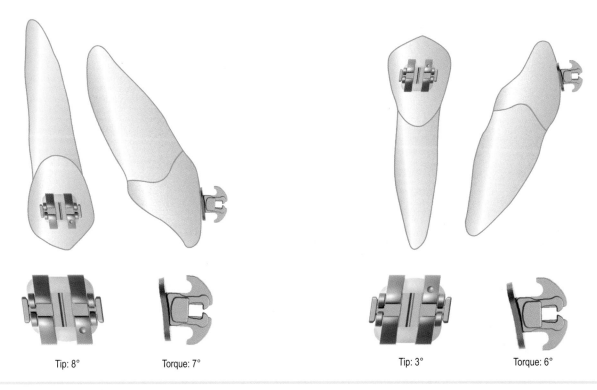

Tip: 8°   Torque: 7°   Tip: 3°   Torque: 6°

Figs 5.15 & 5.16   Versatility – upper canine bracket rotated 180°, providing 8° angulation and +7° torque, and lower canine bracket rotated 180°, providing 3° angulation and +6° torque, positioned on the buccal surface of the respective tooth.

- Protrusive canines: −7° torque for the upper canines and −6° for the lower canines are not recommended in patients with protruding teeth, and when there is gingival recession at the beginning of treatment. In these patients, select brackets with positive torque or neutral torque for the upper and lower canines.

- Extraction cases: zero torque brackets show a tendency to maintain the root of the canines in the alveolar bone, thus facilitating inclination control for these teeth during space closure.

- Deep overbite: in Class II division 2 cases or in deep overbite cases, there is always the need to move the crown of the lower canine buccally and to maintain the root in the center of the alveolar bone. This is easier to achieve when using brackets with 0° or +6° torque for the lower canines.

- Rapid maxillary expansion: expansion of the maxilla is followed by secondary expansion of the lower arch. For these cases, use zero torque or positive torque for the lower canines to support this favorable change.

- Agenesis of upper lateral incisors, when the treatment plan is to close space: when one or both lateral incisors are missing, rotate the bracket on the upper canine by 180°.[1] This procedure changes the torque from −7° to +7°, keeping the same angulation. In these situations, labial crown torque is more appropriate, because the canines occupy the position of the lateral incisors.

Dental arch form

Generally, when patients have well-developed arches, and there is no need to move teeth excessively, −7° brackets for the upper canines and −6° for the lower canines should be used. For ovoid or tapered arches, 0° torque brackets are more appropriate for both the upper and lower canines. When the patient has narrow and tapered arches, +7° brackets for the upper canines and 0° or +6° for the lower canines should be used.

Using the tubes of the lower second/first molars on the upper first and second molars of the opposite side, in cases finishing in a Class II molar relationship

The individual characteristics of the patient should be considered when planning the final position of the teeth. In some cases the treatment plan may dictate a final occlusion with a Class II molar relationship. As a result, it is necessary to adjust the tooth positions to fit this interarch relationship. The average angulation of 5° for Class I upper molars is not appropriate in the Class II relationship. It therefore becomes necessary to customize the position of the upper molar. Ideal positioning of upper molars in a Class II relationship will prevent occlusal interferences during mandibular movements.

Another characteristic of the Class II interarch relationship is mesiolingual rotation of the upper molars. The normal 10° rotation of upper molar tubes is correct for a Class I relationship, but it should not be used when the molars are in a Class II relationship. To obtain 0° rotation for the upper molars with the SmartClip™ Self-Ligating Appliance, second/first lower molar buccal tubes (MBT™ prescription[1]) should be used on the upper molars on the opposite side. As the lower molar tubes have no in-built rotation, the upper molar will present a mesiolingual rotation, occupying more space in the total perimeter of the dental arch. This helps to maintain the contact point in upper premolar extraction cases. Furthermore, this may also be applied in cases of agenesis of upper lateral incisors when the treatment plan requires closing of spaces (Figs 5.17 & 5.18).

Angulation for Class I upper molars

The original Straight-Wire™ Appliance[2] recommends buccal tubes for upper molars with 5° angulation. However, in some cases, this angulation proves to be excessive due to extrusion of the distobuccal cusp of the upper first molars. Results of more recent research studies (Fig. 5.19) verify that the 5° angulation evident

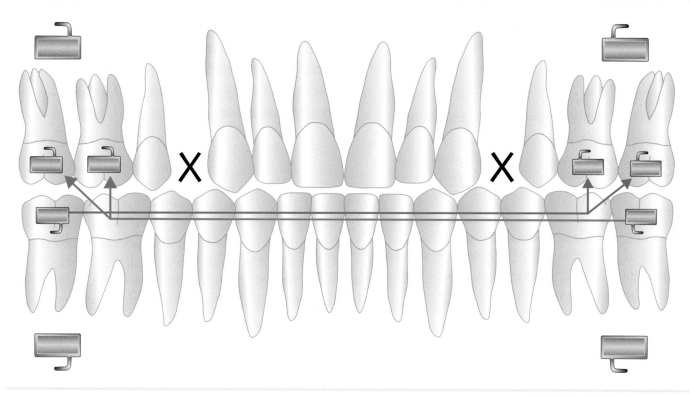

Fig. 5.17 In upper premolar extraction cases, finish the treatment using lower second molar tubes on the upper first and second molars of the opposite side.

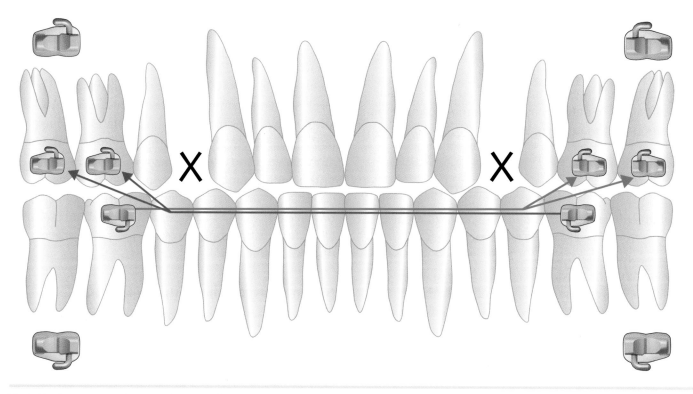

Fig. 5.18 In upper premolar extraction cases, when extra torque control is needed, finish the treatment using lower first molar low profile buccal tubes on the upper first and second molars of the opposite side. This will deliver −20° of buccal root torque.

in natural occlusions is achieved by using upper first molar brackets with 0° angulation in orthodontic cases.

Average angulation for the upper first molar	
Andrews	5.7°
Watanabe	4.5°
Zanelato	5.5°
SWA original	5.0°

Fig. 5.19 Average angulations from research of upper first molars with normal angulation and the prescription of the original Straight-Wire™ Appliance.

With the SmartClip™ Self-Ligating Appliance, as with the MBT™ system, the correct angulation for the molars is obtained using 0° tubes positioned parallel to the buccal intermarginal ridge line (see Chapter 3) (Figs 5.20 & 5.21). In this way 5° of angulation is achieved for the upper first molar crown. If bonding a 5° tube, the mesial portion of the tube should be positioned more toward the gingival to avoid excessive angulation, which could cause extrusion of the distobuccal cusp of the upper first molar and, probably, occlusal interference. Due to the great difference between the maximum and minimum values of tooth angulation in the literature, in some cases the bracket should be repositioned during the finishing stage of treatment if occlusal interferences are present.

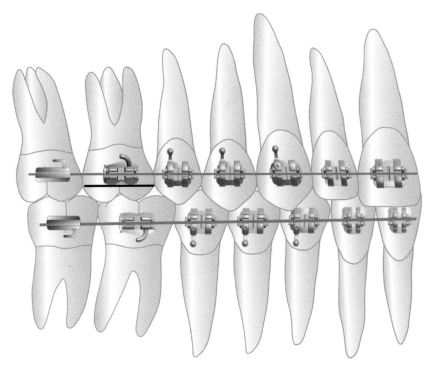

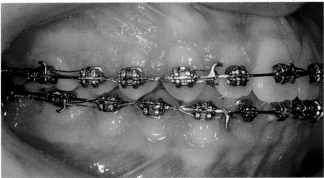

Figs 5.20 & 5.21 Upper first molar tube positioned parallel to the buccal intermarginal ridge line establishing 5° angulation.

Angulation for Class II upper molars

Orthodontic cases in which only upper premolar extractions are planned or cases with agenesis of upper premolars or upper lateral incisors, when the treatment plan is to close space (Figs 5.22, 5.23, 5.24 & 5.25) are finished in Class II molar relationship. In these situations, it is necessary to customize the positioning of the upper molar tubes because the 5° angulation recommended for the Class I relationship is not appropriate for the Class II relationship.[1]

Generally, the upper molars should be upright when finishing the case in Class II. To obtain better occlusion for the lower molars, the upper molar tubes should be positioned with 0° angulation – the long axis of the

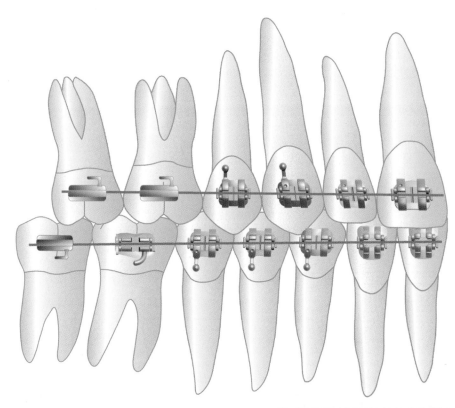

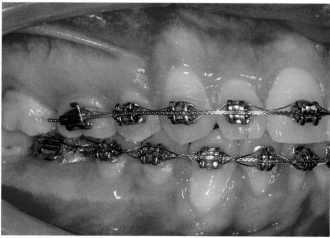

Figs 5.22 & 5.23   Lower left second molar tube on the upper right first molar, when finishing the case in Class II molar relationship (due to the extraction of the premolars). The upper molar should show 0° angulation.

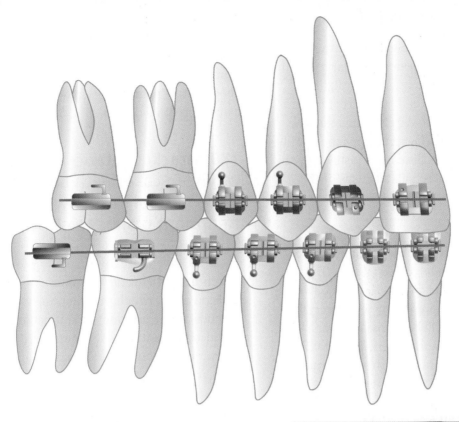

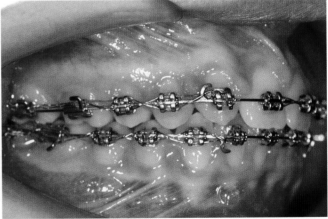

Figs 5.24 & 5.25 Use of the lower left second molar tube on the upper right first molar, when finishing the case in Class II molar relationship (due to the agenesis of the right lateral incisor). The molar should show 0° angulation.

clinical crown should be perpendicular to the occlusal plane.

In Class II cases, the final stage of treatment should receive special attention. In some cases, to obtain the desired angulation for the molars, it is necessary to replace bands with bonded tubes to give a negative

angulation to the crown. The tube should be positioned with −5° angulation to eliminate the 5° natural angulation, uprighting the crown in relation to the occlusal plane (Fig. 5.25). After replacing the bands with bonded buccal tubes, the final archwires will move the root mesially.

Inclination for Class II upper molars

The SmartClip™ Self-Ligating Appliance features the MBT™ value of −14° torque for upper molars. Comparing this value with the original Straight-Wire™ Appliance,[2] the additional buccal root torque is evident (−9° in the Straight-Wire™ Appliance and −14° in the SmartClip™ Self-Ligating Appliance). This increase in crown lingual inclination is justified by the need to avoid extrusion of the palatal cusps of the upper molars, thus preventing possible occlusal interferences.

When applying the versatility of the appliance, tubes of lower second molars can be placed on Class II upper molars, which results in −10° buccal root torque for the upper molars.[1] In cases presenting with buccally inclined second molars, it will be necessary to add bends (torque) in the rectangular archwire or to bond lower first molar low profile tubes with −20° torque to these teeth to achieve better crown position (Fig. 5.26).

Rotation for Class II upper molars

The 10° rotation suggested for Class I upper molars is not appropriate for a Class II molar relationship; instead 0° rotation is recommended.[1] This is achieved by using the tubes of the lower second or first molars

on the upper first and second molars on the opposite side. This helps to move the upper molar crown in a mesiolingual direction. Consequently, these teeth will occupy more space in the dental arch and establish good contact points, especially in upper premolar extraction cases (Figs 5.27 & 5.28).

180° bracket rotation for the upper canine in cases with agenesis of the upper lateral incisor when the treatment plan is to close space

There are several treatment options for cases presenting with agenesis of lateral incisors. The decision about which treatment plan would be best depends on the interarch relationship and the stability of the lower dental arch. When there is a Class I interarch relationship and no need for extraction of lower premolars, the best option is to open anterior spaces for prosthetic rehabilitation. When there is a Class II interarch relationship and the mandibular arch is stable, a good treatment plan is to close spaces, with establishment of a full Class II molar relationship and replacement of the missing lateral incisor with the canine. When there is a Class II interarch relationship and the mandibular arch is unstable, extraction of two

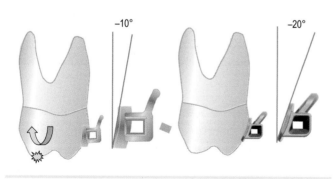

Fig. 5.26 Use of −10° lower second molar tube on the upper first molar with additional torque to overcome occlusal interferences from the palatal cusps; −20° low profile lower first molar tube without additional torque provides a good control of the palatal cusp.

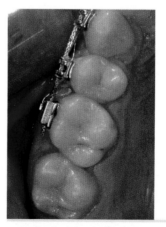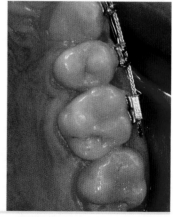

Figs 5.27 & 5.28 End of orthodontic treatment: lower second molar tubes on the upper first molars. The upper first molars do not show rotation, occupying more space in the mesiodistal direction.

lower premolars is recommended, with space closure in the upper arch to obtain a Class I relationship.

As with the MBT™ treatment philosophy, when the treatment plan involves finishing the case to a Class II relationship, with the canines replacing the lateral incisors, two versatility options of the SmartClip Self-Ligating Appliance should be applied:[1]

● Use lower second or first molars tubes on the upper molars on the opposite side, so these teeth will be appropriately positioned in the new occlusal relationship.

● Rotate the canine bracket by 180° so the negative inclination will become positive.

When the canines are going to replace the upper lateral incisors, these teeth should show labial crown inclination. In this way it will be easier to achieve mesial movement of these teeth. The root will move

lingually, thus reducing the contact with the buccal cortical bone, which in this region is very dense due to the presence of the canine buttress of the maxillary bone (Figs 5.29 & 5.30). It is better to use a rotated canine bracket rather than a lateral incisor bracket because the adaptation of the canine bracket to the labial surface of the tooth will be better, and also because these brackets have reduced in–out values.

Interchangeable upper premolar brackets – the same angulation and torque

Brackets for upper premolars feature 0° angulation and –7° torque.[1] The lack of angulation of the upper premolars allows the use of a single bracket for all upper premolars, simplifying the inventory. The use of upper premolar brackets with 0° angulation also reduces anchorage needs and facilitates finishing in a Class I relationship (Figs 5.31 & 5.32).

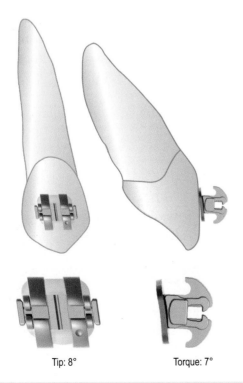

Tip: 8°   Torque: 7°

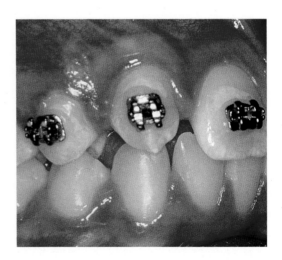

Figs 5.29 & 5.30   In cases of agenesis of lateral incisors, when the treatment plan is to close space, the canine bracket should be positioned rotated 180°, providing 8° angulation and +7° torque.

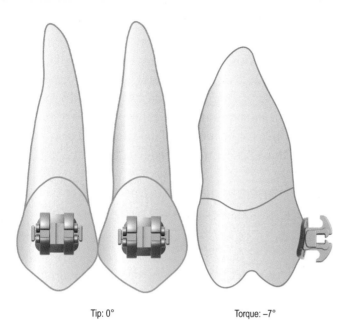

Tip: 0°   Torque: –7°

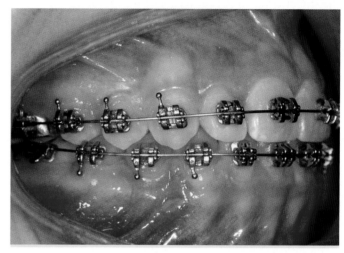

Figs 5.31 & 5.32 Interchangeable upper premolar brackets with 0° angulation and –7° torque.

Interchangeable lower incisor brackets – the same angulation and torque

Brackets for lower incisors feature 0° angulation and –6° torque. The zero angulation of lower incisors is based on results of several studies conducted on normal natural occlusions. Thus, it is possible to use a single bracket for all lower incisors, simplifying the

inventory.[1] With the use of non-angulated brackets for lower incisors, better control of arch length is achieved, preventing the incisor protrusion seen in cases treated using bracket systems with mesial angulation (Figs 5.33 & 5.34).

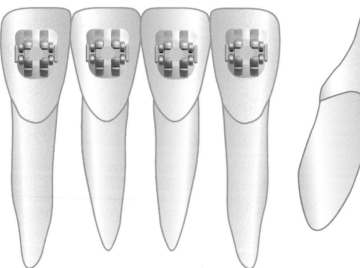

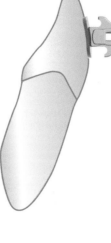

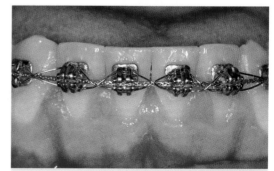

Tip: 0°   Torque: –6°

Figs 5.33 & 5.34 Interchangeable lower incisor bracket with 0° angulation and –6° torque.

References

1. McLaughlin R P, Bennett J C, Trevisi H J 2001 Systemized orthodontic treatment mechanics. Mosby, Edinburgh

2. Andrews L F 1989 Straight-Wire: the concept and appliance. L A Wells, San Diego, p 407

3. Trevisi H J 2005 The SmartClip™ self-ligating appliance system. Technique Guide. 3M Company

4. Bolton W A 1952 Disharmony in tooth size and its relation to the analysis and treatment of malocclusion. Thesis (Master of Science in Dentistry), University of Washington, Seattle, p 40

5. Lischer B E 1911 The diagnosis of malocclusion. Dental Cosmos 53:412–422

6. van der Linden F P G M 1990 Facial growth and facial orthopedics. Quintessence Publishing, New York

7. Zanelato R C, Mandetta S, Gil C T A 2005 Application of the versatility of the MBT™ preadjusted appliance system in cases presenting upper lateral incisor in linguoversion. Revista Dental Press de Ortodontia e Ortopedia Facial 4:52–63

8. McLaughlin R P, Bennett J C 1993 Orthodontic treatment mechanics and the preadjusted appliance. Mosby-Wolfe, London

9. Andrews L F 1972 The six keys to normal occlusion. American Journal of Orthodontics 62:296–309

10. Trevisi Zanelato A C 2003 Evaluation of dental angulation and tipping in Brazilian subjects presenting natural normal occlusion. Thesis (Master Degree in Orthodontics), Methodist University of São Paulo, Brazil

11. Ricketts R M 1976 Bioprogressive therapy as an answer to orthodontics needs Part I. American Journal of Orthodontics 70:241–268

CHAPTER 5 CLINICAL CASE

Name: FF
Sex: Female
Age: 13.5 years
Facial pattern: Brachyfacial
Skeletal pattern: Class I

Diagnosis

A 4 mm Class II malocclusion on the right side and 2 mm Class II malocclusion on the left side, upper midline deviation to the right side, congenitally missing upper right lateral incisor and an accentuated curve of Spee.

Treatment plan

Finish with a Class II molar relationship on the right side and Class I on the left side, with correction of the upper midline, and leveling of the curve of Spee while controlling the inclination of the lower incisors.

Appliance

- SmartClip™ Self-Ligating Appliance
- Apply SmartClip™ Appliance versatility options on upper right canine and first and second molars
- Upper modified Hawley wraparound retainer
- Lower 3–3 fixed retainer

Case report

The patient presented with agenesis of the upper right lateral incisor (tooth 12), a 4 mm Class II malocclusion on the right side, a 2 mm Class II malocclusion on the left side, a 2 mm deviation of upper midline to the right, accentuated curve of Spee, marked labial inclination of the lower incisors and a low mandibular plane as shown by the cephalometric measurements.

The treatment plan was to close the spaces in the upper arch, bringing the right canine into the right lateral

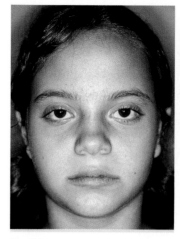
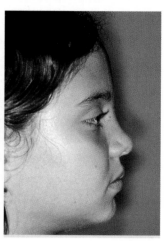

Fig. 5.35   Fig. 5.36

Figs 5.35 & 5.36
Pretreatment photographs showing facial symmetry, Class I profile and good lip seal.

incisor position, correcting the midline, controlling the inclination of the lower incisors to finish in a Class II molar relationship on the right side and a Class I molar relationship on the left side.

Two versatility options of the SmartClip™ Appliance were applied to achieve the treatment aims:

- Use of the lower left second molar tube on the upper right molars to position these teeth without rotation and with 0° angulation.
- Position the upper left canine bracket rotated 180° with the objective of introducing +7° positive torque and maintaining the 8° angulation.

Class III elastics were used on the right side and Class II elastics on the left side to correct the midline. Class III elastics were used with a .018 stainless steel archwire

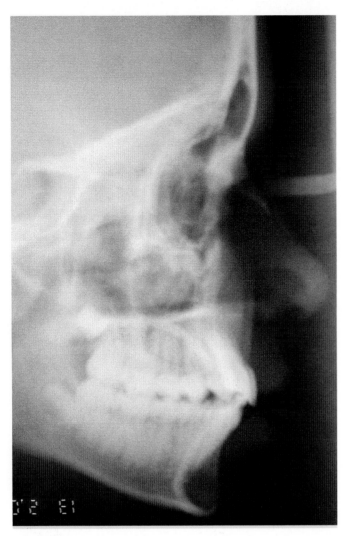

Fig. 5.37

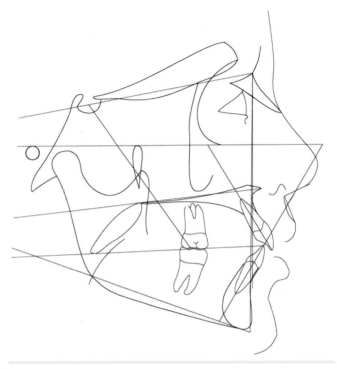

Fig. 5.38

Figs 5.37, 5.38 & 5.39
Pretreatment cephalometric X-ray, tracing and measurements showing a low angle skeletal pattern and increased labial inclination of the lower incisors.

in the lower arch to control the inclination of the lower incisors. Following this a rectangular archwire was used, which imparted buccal root torque to these teeth.

The initial and final cephalometric tracing showed initial IMPA (L1 to Md plane) 102° and final IMPA 101°. The curve of Spee was corrected with good torque control of the lower incisors.

SNA ∠	80°
SNB ∠	79°
ANB ∠	1°
A-N ⊥ FH	0 mm
Po-N ⊥ FH	0 mm
Wits	2 mm
GoGn SN ∠	28°
FH Md ∠	19°
Mx Md ∠	25°
U1 to A-Po	9 mm
L1 to A-Po	5 mm
U1 to Mx plane ∠	116°
L1 to Md plane ∠	102°
Facial analysis	
Nasolabial ∠	91°
NA ⊥ nose	29 mm
Lip thickness	10 mm

Fig. 5.39

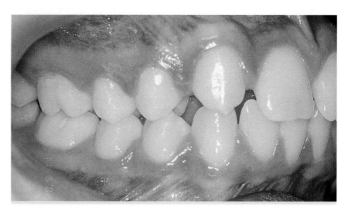

Fig. 5.40

Figs 5.40, 5.41 & 5.42
Pretreatment intraoral photographs showing upper midline deviation to the right side, missing upper right lateral incisor, 4 mm Class II molar relationship on the right side and a 2 mm Class II molar relationship on the left side.

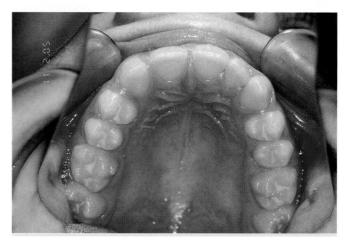

Fig. 5.43

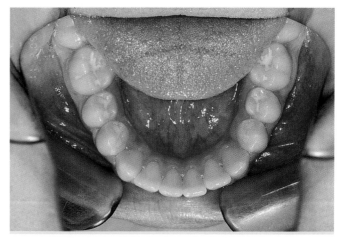

Figs 5.43 & 5.44
Pretreatment upper and lower occlusal views showing good arch form and contour of the upper and lower arches.

Fig. 5.44

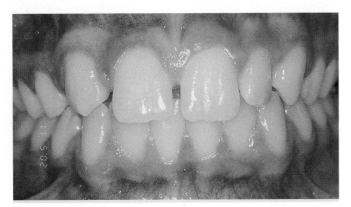

Fig. 5.41

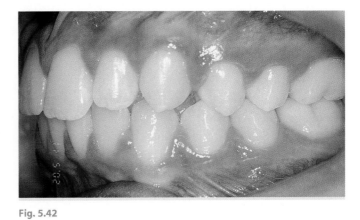

Fig. 5.42

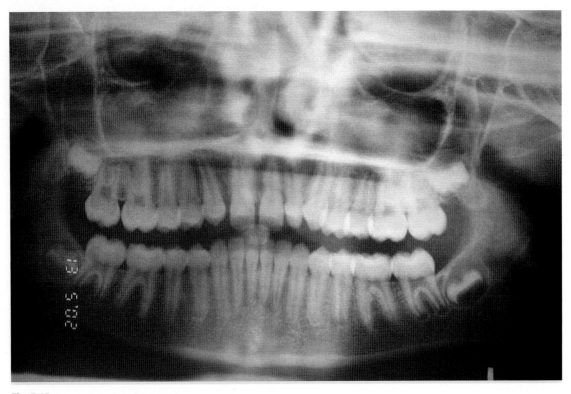

Fig. 5.45

Fig. 5.45
Panoramic X-ray showing full permanent dentition and accentuated curve of Spee.

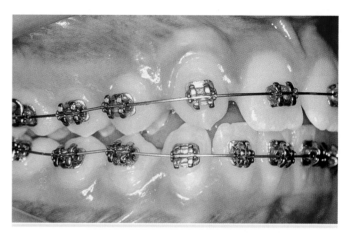

Fig. 5.46

Figs 5.46, 5.47 & 5.48
SmartClip™ Self-Ligating Appliance on the upper and lower arches, with .014 Nitinol round archwire to start aligning. Versatility option applied: upper right canine bracket rotated 180° to provide +7° torque.

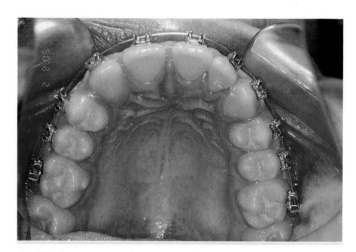

Fig. 5.49

Figs 5.49 & 5.50
Upper and lower occlusal views showing aligning with .014 round Nitinol archwire. In the lower arch, the appliance set-up included the second molars (direct bonding), and in the upper arch, the appliance set-up was up to the first molars (direct bonding). Distal bends were placed in both upper and lower archwires.

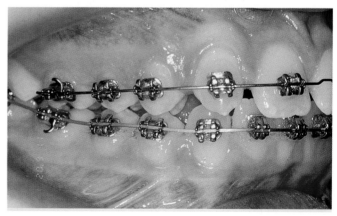

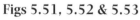

Fig. 5.51

Figs 5.51, 5.52 & 5.53
Leveling with .018 round Nitinol archwire in the upper arch and .017/.025 rectangular Nitinol archwire in the lower arch.

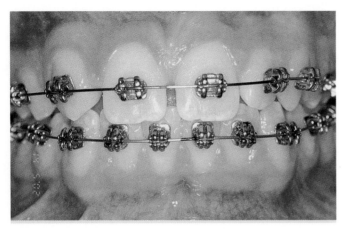

Fig. 5.47

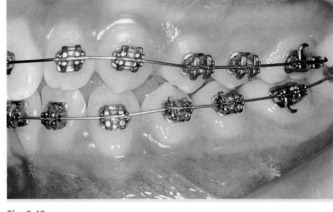

Fig. 5.48

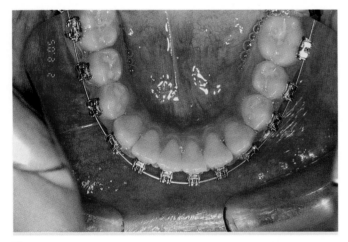

Fig. 5.50

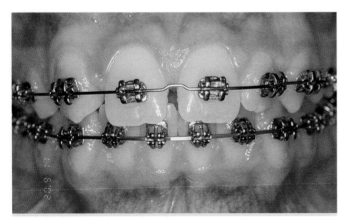

Fig. 5.52

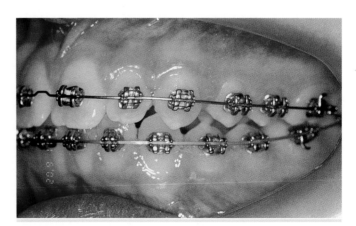

Fig. 5.53

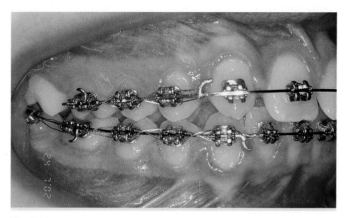

Fig. 5.54

Figs 5.54, 5.55 & 5.56
A .019/.025 stainless steel rectangular archwire in the upper arch, and a .018 stainless steel round archwire in the lower arch with hooks welded mesial to the canines to apply space closure mechanics with use of Class II and Class III elastics.

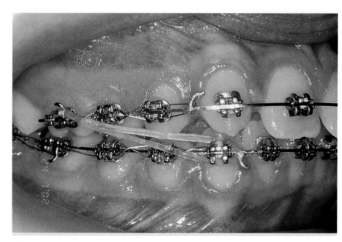

Fig. 5.57

Figs 5.57 & 5.58
Class III elastic used on the right side to encourage loss of anchorage.

Fig. 5.59
SmartClip™ buccal tube for molars, allowing addition of the distal bend before engaging the wire into the bracket slot.

Figs 5.60, 5.61 & 5.62
Occlusal view of the upper right molar with .018 rounded Nitinol archwire and distal bend. Set-up of buccal tube on the upper second molars and re-leveling of the upper arch with a .018 round Nitinol archwire.

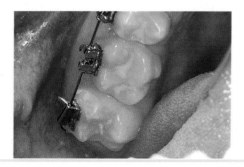

Fig. 5.60

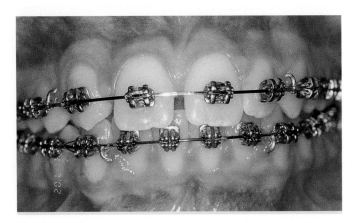

Fig. 5.55

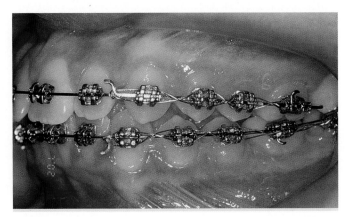

Fig. 5.56

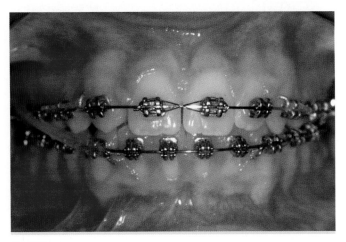

Fig. 5.58

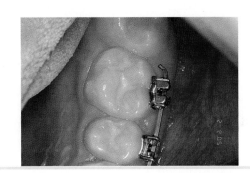

Fig. 5.59

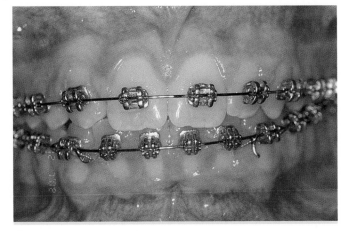

Fig. 5.61

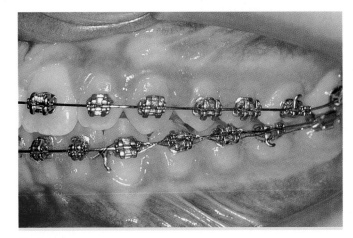

Fig. 5.62

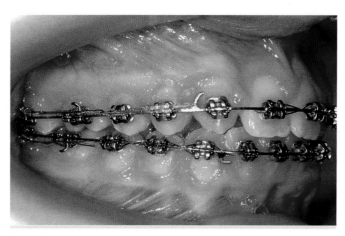

Figs 5.63, 5.64 & 5.65
A .019/.025 stainless steel rectangular archwire on the upper arch and a .018 stainless steel rounded archwire on the lower arch with hooks welded to the mesial of the canines.

Fig. 5.63

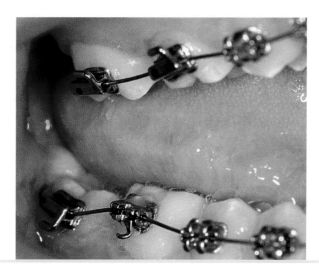

Figs 5.66, 5.67 & 5.68
Application of versatility of the SmartClip™ Appliance for detailing. The lower left second MBT™ molar tubes are bonded on the upper right first and second molars. The lower right first molar tube was repositioned and a .016 round Nitinol archwire engaged in both arches.

Fig. 5.66

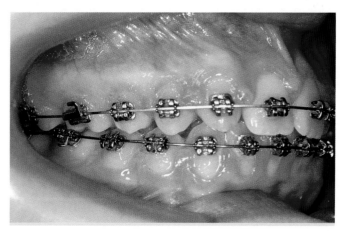

Figs 5.69, 5.70 & 5.71
A .019/.025 rectangular Nitinol archwire in the upper arch and a .018 stainless steel round archwire in the lower arch at the end of the detailing stage.

Fig. 5.69

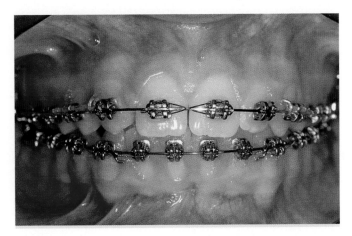

Fig. 5.64

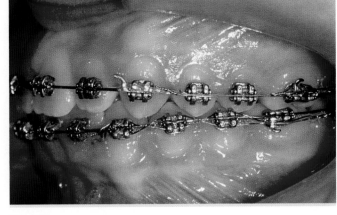

Fig. 5.65

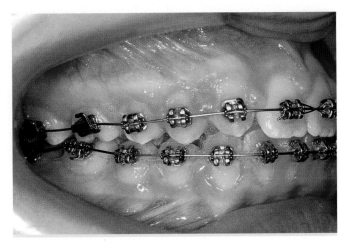

Fig. 5.67

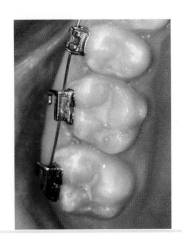

Fig. 5.68

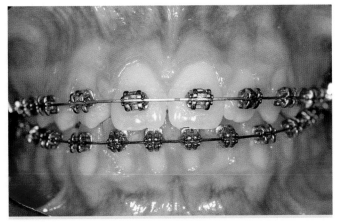

Fig. 5.70

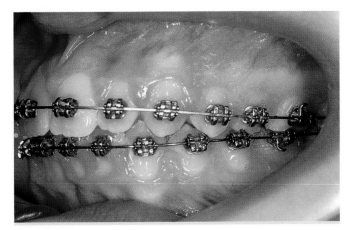

Fig. 5.71

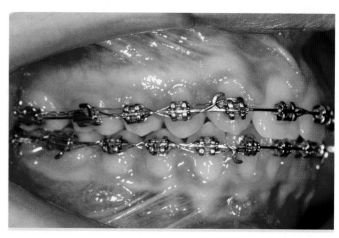

Fig. 5.72

Figs 5.72, 5.73 & 5.74
Final stage of finishing and detailing with .019/.025 stainless steel rectangular archwires in the upper and lower arches.

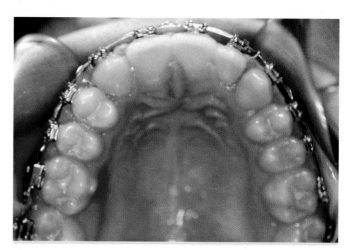

Fig. 5.75

Figs 5.75 & 5.76
Final stage of treatment. Upper and lower occlusal views showing the arch form and alignment of the teeth in both arches.

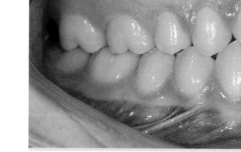

Fig. 5.77

Figs 5.77, 5.78 & 5.79
Post-treatment intraoral photographs showing Class II occlusion on the right side, Class I on the left side and corrected midline.

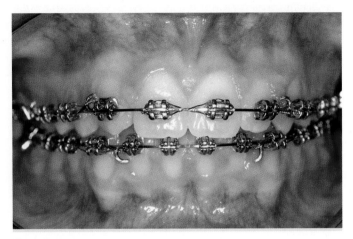

Fig. 5.73

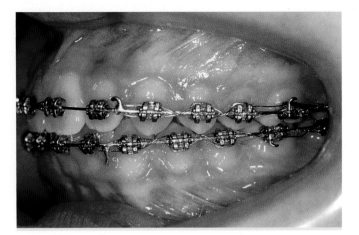

Fig. 5.74

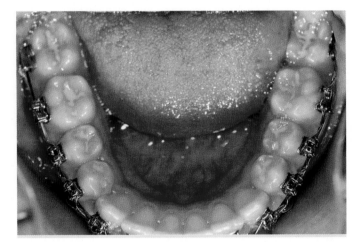

Fig. 5.76

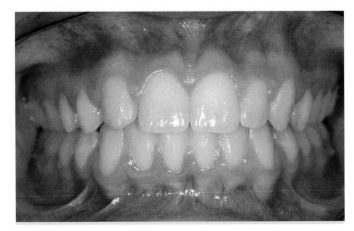

Fig. 5.78

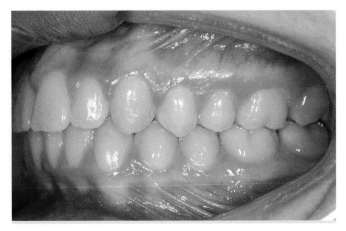

Fig. 5.79

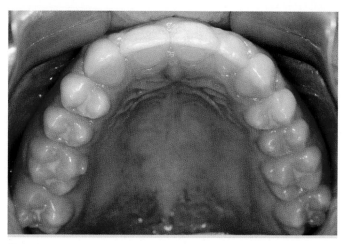

Figs 5.80, 5.81 & 5.82
Post-treatment upper and lower occlusal views
showing a 3–3 fixed retainer on the lower arch, and
anterior guidance view.

Fig. 5.80

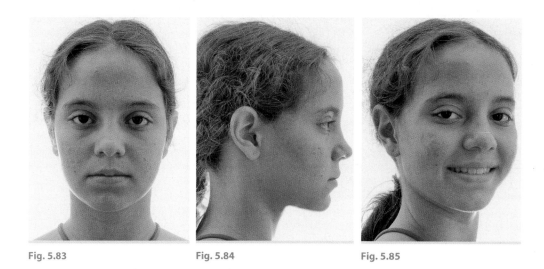

Fig. 5.83   Fig. 5.84   Fig. 5.85

Figs 5.83, 5.84 & 5.85
Post-treatment photographs showing facial symmetry, Class I facial profile, good lip
seal and good smile line.

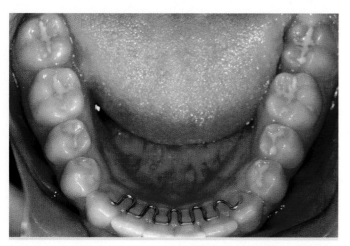

Fig. 5.81

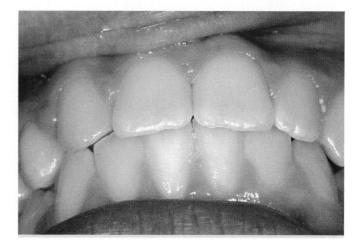

Fig. 5.82

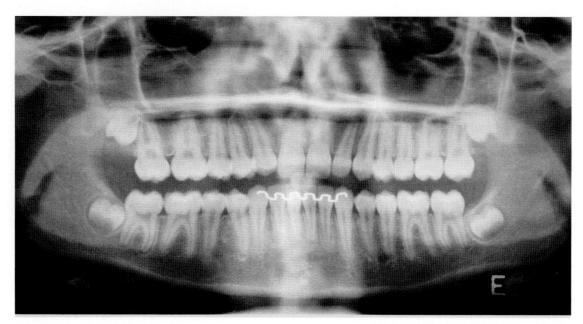

Fig. 5.86

Fig. 5.86
Panoramic X-ray showing root parallelism and the upper right canine positioned in the place of the lateral incisor.

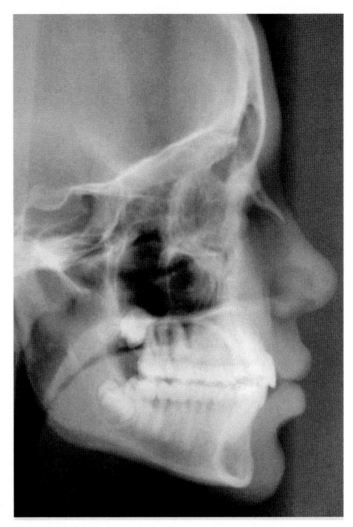

Fig. 5.87, 5.88, 5.89 & 5.90
Post-treatment cephalometric X-ray, tracing and measurements showing good torque control of the lower incisors at the end of treatment. Superimposition of the initial and final cephalometric tracings shows good growth and torque control of the lower incisors.

Fig. 5.87

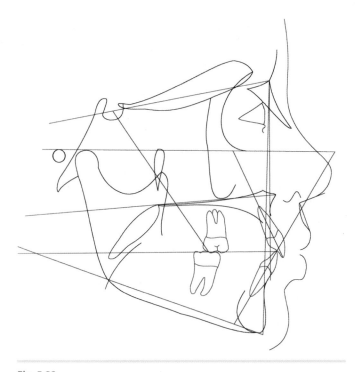

Fig. 5.88

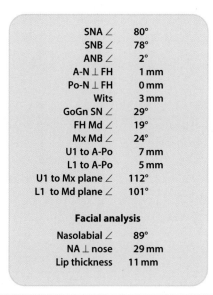

SNA ∠	80°
SNB ∠	78°
ANB ∠	2°
A-N ⊥ FH	1 mm
Po-N ⊥ FH	0 mm
Wits	3 mm
GoGn SN ∠	29°
FH Md ∠	19°
Mx Md ∠	24°
U1 to A-Po	7 mm
L1 to A-Po	5 mm
U1 to Mx plane ∠	112°
L1 to Md plane ∠	101°

Facial analysis

Nasolabial ∠	89°
NA ⊥ nose	29 mm
Lip thickness	11 mm

Fig. 5.89

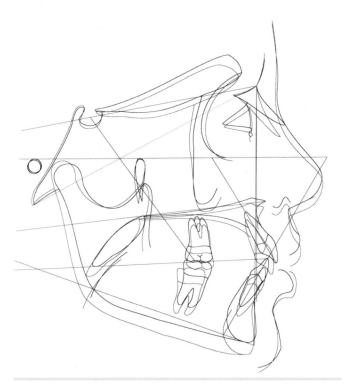

Fig. 5.90

CHAPTER 6

Occlusion in orthodontics

Introduction

The main objective of this chapter is to discuss the stomatognathic system, focusing on important factors such as centric occlusion, functional movements, orthopedically stable position of the condyles in the mandibular fossae, and the interrelationship of these factors during orthodontic treatment. The teeth play a major part in the functioning of the stomatognathic system, and orthodontic treatment should aim to position the teeth in the mandibular and maxillary bones such that they establish an optimal relationship with neighboring and antagonist teeth, leading to a functionally balanced occlusion. Careful diagnosis and treatment planning, and correct application of mechanics and techniques can help clinicians provide a functionally balanced orthodontic treatment result with good facial esthetics.

The SmartClip™ Self-Ligating Appliance[1] has the same tip and torque specifications as the MBT™ system,[2] and by means of its angulation, torque, rotation, .022/.028 slot, and the use of .019/.025 rectangular archwires, allows optimal execution of sliding mechanics and conclusion of the orthodontic treatment with the teeth well positioned in both jaws. Thus the SmartClip™ Self-Ligating Appliance includes all the features of a preadjusted appliance system that are needed to achieve the goals for a good functional occlusion, occlusion in centric relation and adequate functional movements.

This chapter also discusses the contribution of torque and angulation of each tooth type to centric occlusion and functional movements with respect to a mutually protected occlusion. As has been already mentioned in Chapter 3, individualized positioning of brackets is an important element in obtaining a functional and balanced occlusion following orthodontic treatment. The appliance set-up described in this chapter takes into consideration the dynamics of the patient's occlusion at the end of the orthodontic treatment. It should be recognized that the choice of the appliance and the versatility of the technique are critical for detailing the occlusion and achieving the functional goals of orthodontic treatment.

The ability of the mandible to move in all three dimensions often makes it difficult to understand how teeth occlude and disclude during the various movements. However, occlusion and disclusion of teeth can affect mandibular movement and the neuromuscular functioning of the temporomandibular joint (TMJ). At the same time, the direction or path of condylar movements, which is determined by the shape of the mandibular fossae and the articular eminence of both joints, influences tooth contact during movements and thus the harmony between the various organizational elements of the occlusion.

Maxillomandibular relationships

Mandibular posture and dynamics significantly influence all functions of the stomatognathic system – mastication, phonation, deglutition, respiration and facial expression. Maxillomandibular relationships can be classified into **static relationships** and **dynamic relationships**.

Static maxillomandibular relationships

The maxillomandibular relationship is described as static when the mandible is not moving in relation to the base of the skull, that is, there is no mandibular movement in any direction. There are four static mandibular positions: postural position, centric relation position, centric occlusion position and centric relation occlusion.

Postural position (resting position)

In this position, the mandible is held suspended by the elevator muscles, whether the patient is in a standing or sitting position. The postural position, also called resting position, is characterized by the relative passivity of the muscles involved and a lack of occlusal contact. The interocclusal space in this position is called phonetic or free functional space and it varies from 2.0 mm to 4.0 mm in the molar region[3] (Fig. 6.1). This position is particularly important in orthodontics,

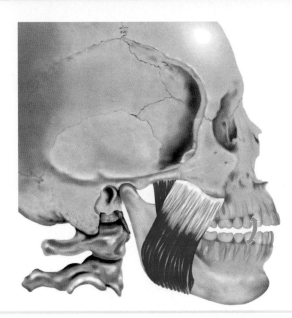

Fig. 6.1 Postural position is determined by the myotactic reflex, and the mandible is suspended by the elevator muscles. Tooth contact should not occur in this position.

because, even during adolescence, individuals often have parafunctional habits such as tooth clenching, associated with pain, muscular discomfort and an inability to maintain the postural position over a period of time. Such individuals routinely keep their teeth in the intercuspation position most of the time. This is unphysiologic and can interfere with orthodontic treatment mechanics.

Centric relation position

The centric relation position has been studied for decades and, from time to time, new definitions have been proposed. More recently, in the late 1980s, a consensus was reached regarding the most suitable definition for this position. In 1998, Jeffrey Okeson[4] suggested a change in the definition of this position, keeping in mind the variety of definitions that had already been proposed. He introduced the term 'orthopedically stable articular position' and defined centric relation as the **mandibular position in which the condyles assume a superoanterior position within the mandibular fossa, resting against the posterior aspect of the articular eminence with the articular disk interposed in between** (Fig. 6.2).

Regardless of the terms given to the position, it is important that orthodontists consider it as a major reference (see below), because of occlusal changes that may occur during treatment.

Methods for taking records in centric relation position

The centric relation position serves as a guide for clinicians in the same way as a lighthouse does for the navigator of a ship. It represents a reference point which the clinician can use to evaluate whether:

1. the diagnosis was correct
2. the treatment plan is appropriate
3. the treatment mechanics have been applied satisfactorily
4. the requirements of functional occlusion have been achieved at the end of treatment
5. the orthopedic components are in harmony with the dental components
6. the treatment is progressing favorably.

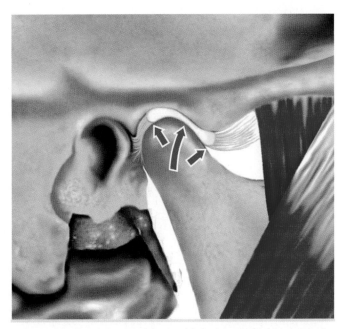

Fig. 6.2 Correct positioning of the condyle in the articular fossa in centric relation position. Superoanterior position with the articular disk properly interposed in between.

The centric relation position can be checked by the clinician at any stage of the orthodontic treatment either directly on the patient by manipulation (Figs 6.3, 6.4, 6.5 & 6.6) or indirectly, with the use of semi- adjustable articulators (Fig. 6.7). Despite assuring the patient that clinical assessment is quicker and involves fewer procedures, a reliable clinical assessment of centric relation can be difficult in some patients due to

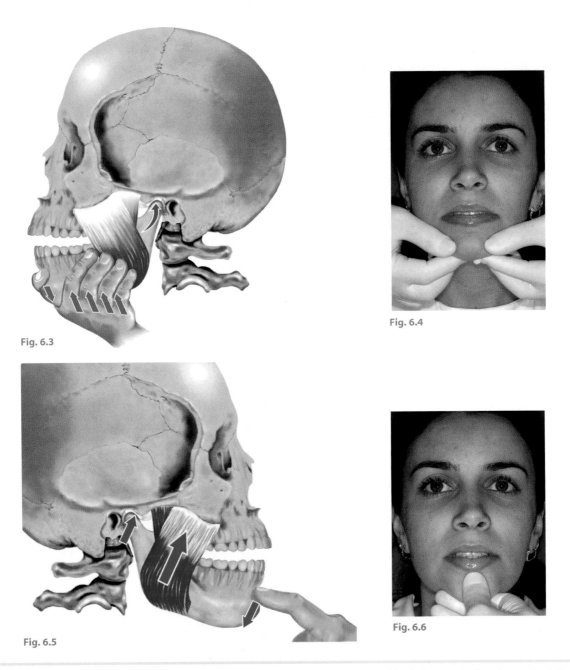

Fig. 6.3

Fig. 6.4

Fig. 6.5

Fig. 6.6

Figs 6.3, 6.4, 6.5 & 6.6 Use of the Dawson bilateral manipulation to correctly position the condyles in the articular fossa in centric relation position. The clinician should move the condyles anterior and superiorly by applying a downward force on the menton with the thumb and at the same time applying upward force on the base of the mandible with the remaining fingers. In the Anderson and Turner menton guiding method, while the clinician's thumb applies a downward force on the menton, generating resistance to the elevation of the mandible, the elevator muscles contract, leading to an anterior and superior positioning of the condyle.

pain or muscular dysfunction or even due to the patient's inability to relax the muscles (Fig. 6.8).

There is an established sequence for indirectly determining the centric relation position. First, the mandibular closure reflex must be deprogrammed to allow relaxation of the masticatory muscles. The use of deprogramming intraoral devices, such as the Victor Lucia jig and Long gauging bands, also known as **leaf gauges**, is advocated by many clinicians and has been shown to obtain the necessary relaxation (Fig. 6.9). When one of these devices is placed between the anterior teeth, the posterior teeth disclude so that the mandible is supported at three points: the TMJs and the anterior deprogamming device. The action of the elevator muscles on both sides positions each condyle–disk complex in a more anatomically balanced position, also called the centric relation position (Fig. 6.10). Besides positioning the condyles, anterior deprogramming devices facilitate taking interocclusal records in centric relation position, as the posterior teeth are not in contact when taking the records (Fig. 6.11). The bite record is taken in centric relation for the purpose of relating the lower model to the upper model on the semi-adjustable articulator, to assist in orthodontic treatment planning and analysis (Figs 6.12 & 6.13).

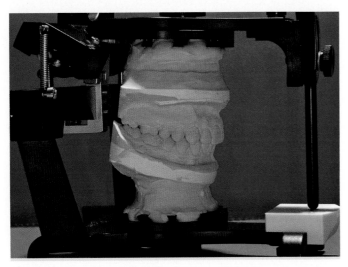

Fig. 6.7   A semi-adjustable articulator can be useful during orthodontic planning.

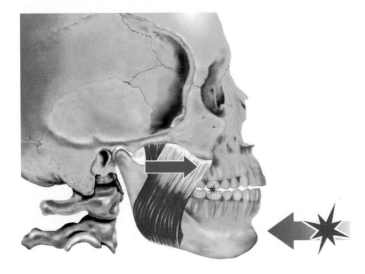

Fig. 6.8   Contraction of the lateral pterygoid muscle can compromise clinical manipulation of the condylar position in centric relation.

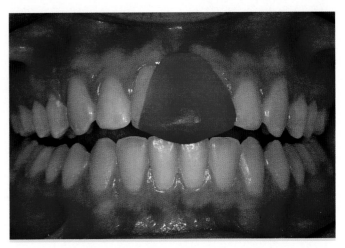

Fig. 6.9   An anterior deprogramming device for obtaining centric relation position – Victor Lucia jig.

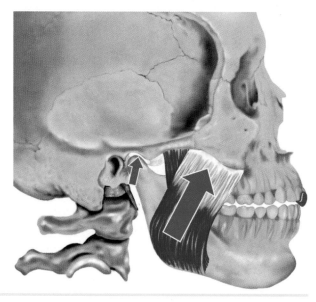

Fig. 6.10 Anterior deprogramming devices provide an anterior stop and allow the elevator muscles to position the condyles anterosuperiorly, in other words, in a more stable position.

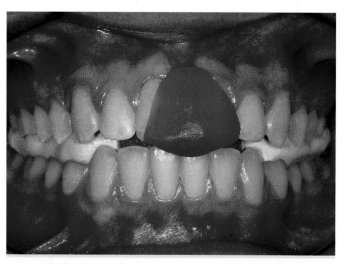

Fig. 6.11 Taking interocclusal records for articulation of models with the anterior deprogramming device.

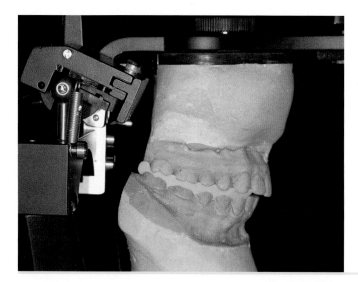

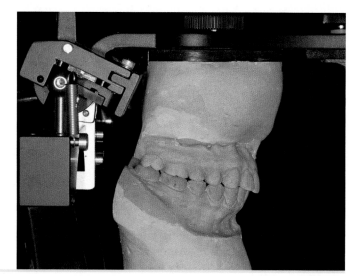

Figs 6.12 & 6.13 Models made of silicone in centric relation with and after removal of the bite record.

Maximal intercuspation position (centric occlusion position)

Centric occlusion refers to an exclusively dental relationship, in which the mandibular posterior teeth are in maximum occlusal contact with their maxillary antagonists at the conclusion of mandibular elevation. Therefore, this is also called the maximal intercuspation position (Figs 6.14, 6.15 & 6.16).

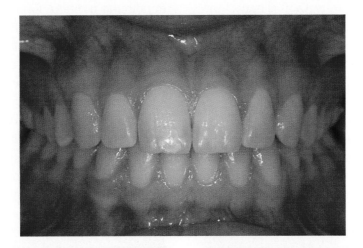

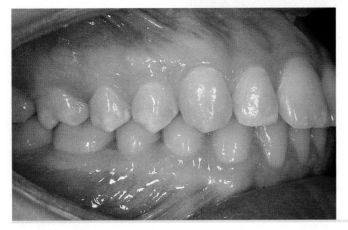
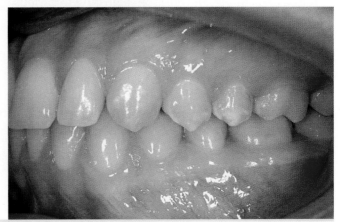

Figs 6.14, 6.15 & 6.16   Frontal and lateral views of the centric occlusion or maximal intercuspation position.

The dental occlusion interrupts mandibular elevation, and at the time of contact the force generated by the elevator muscles must be distributed over all the posterior teeth in a balanced way, via simultaneous bilateral contact. In this position, the incisal edges of the mandibular anterior teeth should be free of any contact, although they can lightly touch the palatal surfaces of the maxillary anterior teeth. It is important that the incisal edges of the maxillary and mandibular teeth are in close proximation so that they can provide anterior guidance when the mandible moves away from this position.

During mandibular elevation with the condyles in centric relation position, when initial tooth contact occurs, the neuromuscular system promptly stimulates muscular action with the purpose of positioning the mandible such that there is a more stable occlusal relationship between the antagonist teeth (Fig. 6.17). This explains why centric occlusion is considered an acquired and changeable position, adjusting to various alterations that take place in an individual occlusion throughout their life. Most of these are the result of dental procedures ranging from fissure sealants, to restorations, extractions, and prosthetic and orthodontic treatment.

It is important to know about and to be able to analyze mandibular positions for an accurate diagnosis and treatment plan. When clinicians plan orthodontic treatment, they should not solely rely on the dental relationships displayed on the study models. Although this relationship may correspond to that observed in the patient, the clinician must keep in mind that the mandible may have been in an atypical position as a result of malpositioned teeth or contacts. Functional anterior and posterior crossbites are examples of such cases, as is the patient who presents with a Class I molar relationship but with condyles excessively displaced from the centric relation position (and should be classified as having what could be called a false Class I) (Figs 6.18 & 6.19).

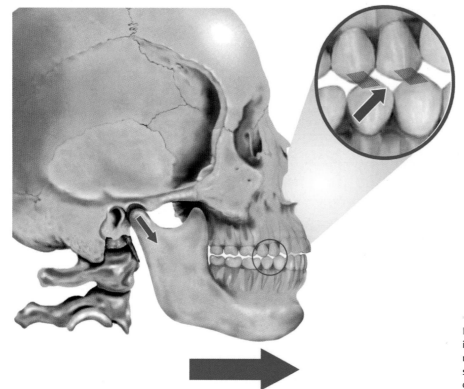

Fig. 6.17 Any dental contact that causes occlusal instability during mandibular elevation in centric relation position can activate the neuromuscular system leading to better distribution of dental contacts.

At the completion of treatment, the centric relation position serves as an important reference for the final evaluation of the orthodontic result. Once all the teeth have moved during the treatment, the clinician loses track of the intercuspation position that the patient showed before treatment. Only the centric relation position is left as a reference for the maxillomandibular relationship. Thus, after completion of treatment, teeth should intercuspate with the condyles positioned as close as possible to the centric relation position.[5]

Centric relation occlusion

Centric relation occlusion occurs when centric relation and centric occlusion, or maximal intercuspation, coincide. Although it could be considered as an ideal clinical outcome, it is not often found even among individuals with naturally normal occlusions. In 1952, Posselt[6] reported that only 10% of the population showed this relationship, and a discrepancy between the two positions occurred in the remaining 90%. However, despite this lack of coincidence between centric condylar position and centric occlusion in individuals with naturally normal occlusions and not necessarily being an indication for treatment, centric relation occlusion represents one of the desirable outcomes for achieving a functional occlusion at the end of orthodontic treatment.

Dynamic maxillomandibular relationships

The dynamic maxillomandibular relationship refers to the functional movements of the mandible, and is further determined by the anatomic characteristics of the TMJs and the neuromuscular system. Mandibular movements occur in complex three-dimensional patterns, depending on the function that the mandible is required to fulfill at that given moment.

The orthodontist should keep in mind that the masticatory cycle combines complex movements of the mandible, which vary according to the type of food – size, shape, hardness, and consistency – and are determined by neural patterns in the central nervous system. In addition, occlusal factors can also influence these movements, and these vary from person to person. This makes comprehension and study of these infinite movements very complicated. Therefore, for didactic reasons, the following less complex and easy to understand method of classification of movements has been adopted in this chapter:

1. Elevation/depression
2. Protrusion/retrusion
3. Right/left lateroprotrusion.

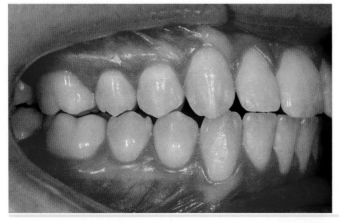 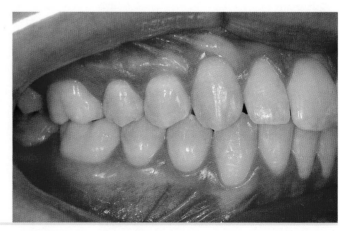

Figs 6.18 & 6.19   Examples of Class I occlusions with condyles *not* in centric relation position.

Mandibular depression

Mandibular depression occurs during opening of the mouth, which is divided into two stages for ease of understanding, depending on the type of movement brought about by the condyles:

● First stage: rotation
● Second stage: translation.

When the condyles are in centric relation position, mandibular depression occurs as a simple rotational movement around an imaginary horizontal axis passing through the center of rotation of both condyles (Figs 6.20, 6.21 & 6.22). Usually this movement takes place until there is a space of between 13 mm and 25 mm between the antagonist central incisors.[7]

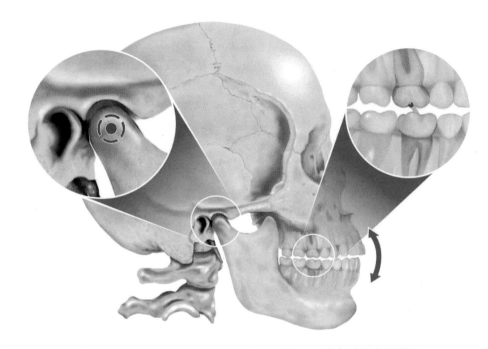

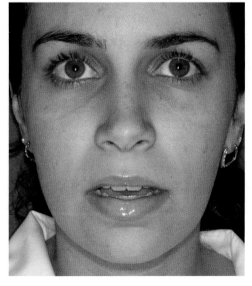
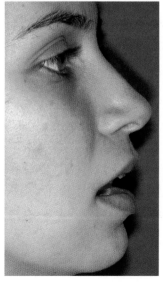

Figs 6.20, 6.21 & 6.22 Condylar rotation occurs when the condyles are within the limits of the mandibular fossae. Clinically, incisal opening of between 13 mm and 25 mm is observed.

The clinical relevance of the space between the incisors is to do with to all the records and adjustment procedures that might need to be carried out in the centric relation position. Remember that if the patient opens the mouth beyond the above mentioned interval, the condyles will be displaced to a more anterior position, thus initiating the second stage of mandibular depression, that is, condylar translation.

As the mandible is depressed beyond the limit of condylar rotation, the condyles begin to slide anteriorly along the articular eminences, until maximal mouth opening is achieved (Figs 6.23, 6.24 & 6.25).

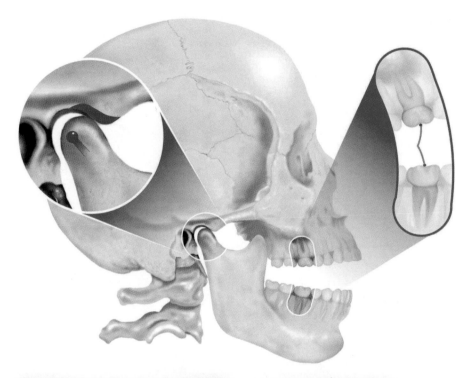

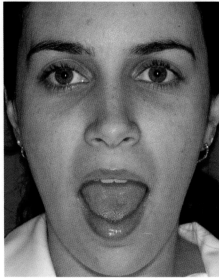

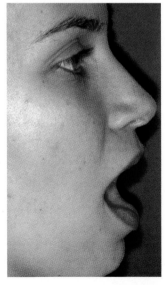

Figs 6.23, 6.24 & 6.25 Beyond the limit of the rotation movement, there is translation of the condyles until maximum mouth opening.

Mandibular elevation

The movement in the direction opposite to mandibular depression is mandibular elevation, which occurs as a result of contraction of the elevator muscles and is completed when the teeth intercuspate.

During elevation, the mandible acts as a class III lever (Figs 6.26 & 6.27). This represents the ideal functional set-up for the masticatory system because it transmits less load to the teeth and attached structures.

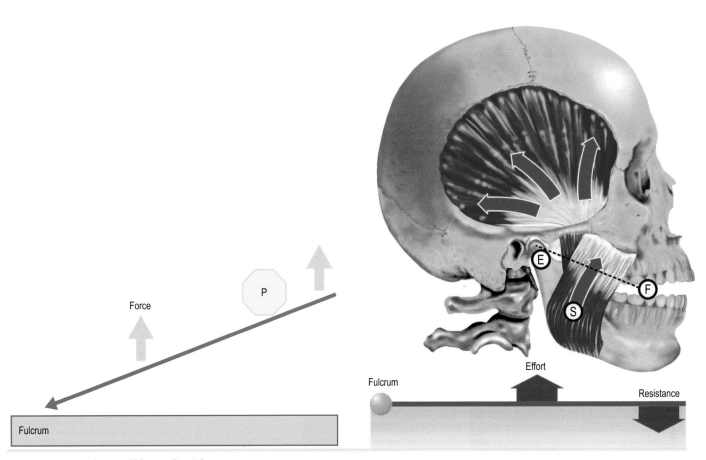

Figs 6.26 & 6.27 The mandible as a class III lever.

According to Okeson,[4] the same force generated by the elevator muscles leads to greater loads on the posterior teeth and lesser loads on the anterior teeth (Figs 6.28 & 6.29). Thus, taking into consideration the distribution of the forces generated by the powerful elevator muscles during mandibular elevation, one can conclude that the anterior teeth have a mechanical advantage in this system.

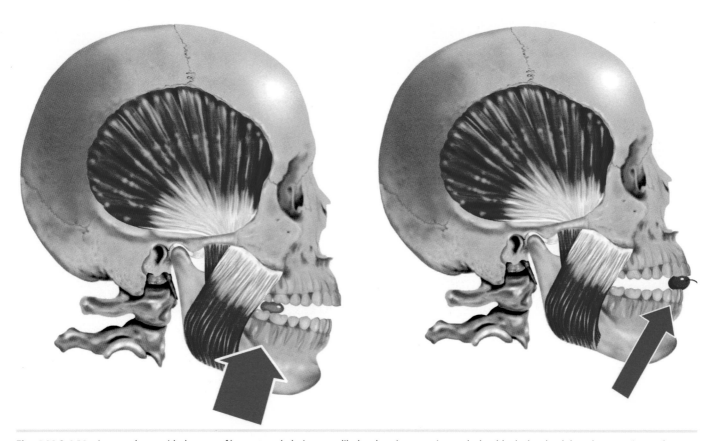

Figs 6.28 & 6.29　In accordance with the type of lever at work during mandibular elevation, anterior teeth should take less load than the posterior teeth.

Mandibular protrusion

The anterior movement of the mandible from the centric occlusal position, with translation of both condyles and disclusion of posterior teeth, is called protrusive movement or protrusion (Figs 6.30 & 6.31). Disclusion of posterior teeth occurs not only due to condylar movement, but also due to the sliding of the lower incisors against the palatal surfaces of the upper teeth (Fig. 6.32). During protrusion, the disclusion of the posterior teeth is important for maintaining the integrity of these teeth and their supporting

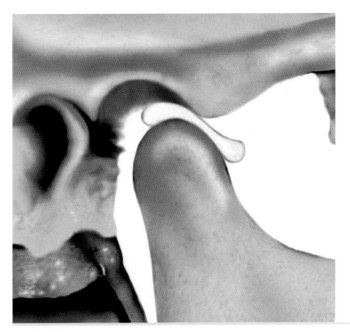
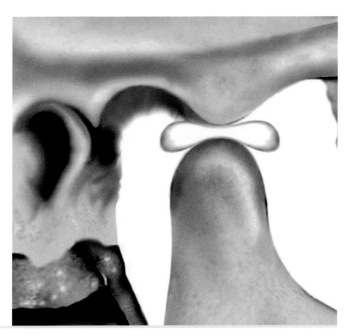

Figs 6.30 & 6.31   During protrusive movement, both condyles move down the posterior walls of the articular eminences, leading to disclusion of the posterior teeth.

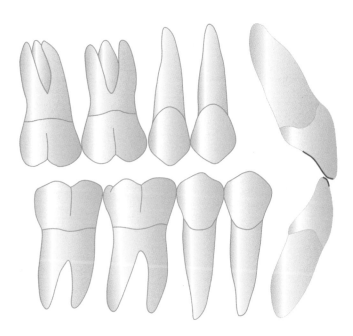

Fig. 6.32   During protrusion, the lower incisors slide down the palatal concavity of the upper incisors, helping with disclusion of the posterior teeth.

periodontal structures, as the horizontal forces generated during this movement are potentially traumatic to these teeth.

For protrusion to take place, some events must occur in a coordinated fashion; in other words, both the inferior lateral pterygoid muscles must contract at the same time as the elevator muscles to maintain the contact between the anterior teeth. This muscular action forces the two condyles downward and forward, along the inclination of the articular eminence. The movement of the condyles results in movement of the entire mandible and, at the same time, the incisal edges of the mandibular anterior teeth slide down the palatal

surfaces of the maxillary anterior teeth from centric occlusion to the edge-to-edge position. This factor leads to a forward and downward bodily movement of the mandible, resulting in disclusion of the posterior teeth (Fig. 6.33).

The above discussion leads us to two important concepts in occlusion: **anterior guidance** and **condylar guidance**. Anterior guidance can be defined as the relationship between the incisal edges of the mandibular anterior teeth and the palatal surfaces of the maxillary anterior teeth during protrusive movement, with disclusion of the posterior teeth (Fig. 6.34). The efficiency of the anterior guidance depends

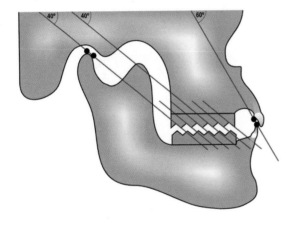

Fig. 6.33 Disclusion of the posterior teeth during protrusive movement is the result of both the translation of the condyles and the dynamic relationship between the upper and lower incisors.

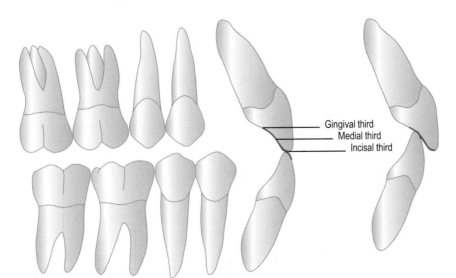

Gingival third
Medial third
Incisal third

Fig. 6.34 Anterior guidance plays an important part in the disclusion of the posterior teeth.

on the overjet and the overbite of the anterior teeth, which directly influence the angulation and height of the anterior guidance (Figs 6.35, 6.36 & 6.37). Condylar guidance is determined by the height and inclination of the posterior slope of the articular eminence (Figs 6.30 & 6.31).

Clinically, anterior guidance is evaluated starting from the intercuspation position, centric occlusion or centric relation occlusion to the edge-to-edge position between the upper central incisors and all the lower incisors. This movement occurs in the opposite direction to the functional movement that occurs when incising food. However, any interference or lack of balance in either direction will also be present during the movement in the opposite direction (Fig. 6.38). The teeth participating in anterior guidance (i.e. the upper central incisors, and sometimes the upper lateral

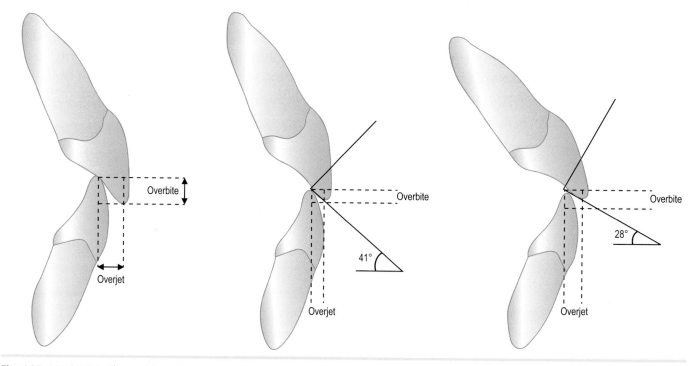

Figs 6.35, 6.36 & 6.37 The overbite and the overjet affect the anterior guidance.

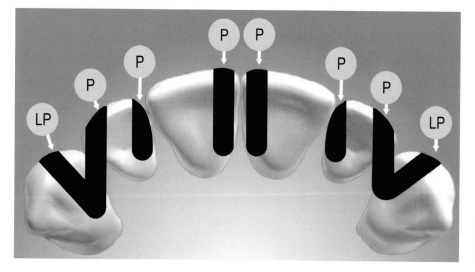

Fig. 6.38 The path of anterior guidance should be clear of interferences in any direction of movement of the mandible.

incisors, and the four lower incisors) benefit from the Class III lever system (see above). As this lever system reduces the loads inflicted on these teeth, the contact between these teeth during the excursive movements of the mandible has very low traumatogenic potential.

Lateroprotrusion

Lateroprotrusion is defined as the lateral movement of the mandible from centric occlusion, until the canines on the side to which the mandible is being moved reach the edge-to-edge position. As in protrusion, a protective mechanism prevents the posterior teeth from contacting during lateral movement. In the case of lateroprotrusion, the canines serve as the movement guides, avoiding interferences between the posterior teeth. This mechanism is called canine guidance (Figs 6.39 & 6.40).

The protection provided by canine guidance is very important for the integrity of the supporting tissues of the posterior teeth, because occlusal interferences

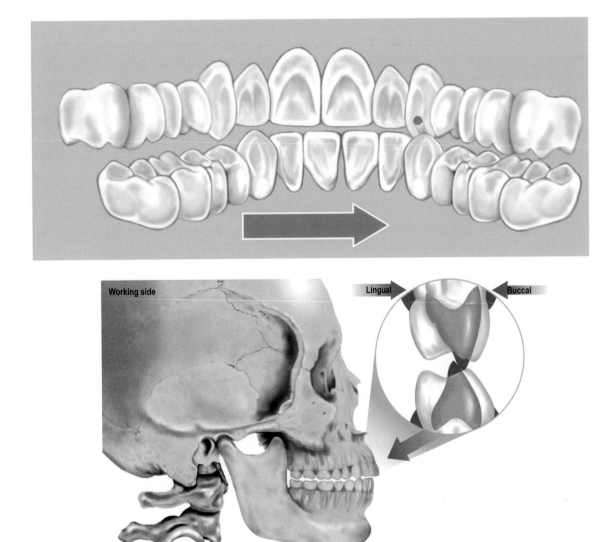

Figs 6.39 & 6.40   The canine guidance should be active during lateroprotrusive movements to avoid any interference between the posterior teeth. During all lateral movements, the canines should contact before the posterior teeth. P, protrusion; LP, lateroprotrusion.

during lateroprotrusive movements can be markedly destructive. If interferences occur during protrusion, the force is delivered in the anteroposterior direction, which may be absorbed and neutralized by the proximal contacts between the teeth. In lateroprotrusion, any type of interference will generate a force which, if applied to the posterior teeth in the buccolingual direction in the absence of a mechanism to oppose this force, will be sufficient to overload the contacting teeth. If this excess load surpasses the structural tolerance limit of the teeth and the periodontal tissues, it can manifest clinically as attrition of the cusp tips, enamel cracks, non-carious cervical lesions, tooth mobility and gingival recession – all of which are often encountered in daily clinical practice. Therefore, to avoid these sequelae, special attention needs to be given to the correct positioning of the canines on the same side. In intercuspation position, the lower canine cusp tip must be as close as possible to the palatal surface of the upper canine, so that at any sign of mandibular lateral movement, the canines on the working side can produce immediate disclusion of the posterior teeth.

D'Amico[8] studied primitive and modern dentitions of humans and animals and defended the concept of an occlusion protected by the canines. From his observations he came to the following conclusions:

● The human dentition was designed for mastication of an omnivorous diet.
● The TMJs provide sliding joint movement, and the position of the condyles in the mandibular fossae is determined by dental contact.
● The canines serve to guide the mandible during eccentric movements in which the antagonist teeth do not make functional contact.
● The contact between the upper and the lower canines determines the lateral movements of the mandible. Canine guidance helps avoid any type of force being applied to the incisors and the posterior teeth.
● The canines are extremely sensitive teeth and, when in contact during eccentric movements, the high

levels of periodontal proprioceptive stimulation reflexively reduce muscular tension and, consequently, the magnitude of the force applied.

Lateroprotrusion is the main movement of the masticatory cycle. This is because the lateral movement of the mandible makes it possible for the teeth to hold the bolus of food. Thus the mandible moves toward the side on which mastication is taking place – for this reason this side is called the **working side**. The opposite side – from which the mandible is heading – is called the **non-working side**.

After the mouth is opened, the mandible (which normally moves straight down in the midline) translates to the working side, the right or the left, and begins to elevate with food between the posterior teeth. These teeth are in edge-to-edge position, heading toward intercuspation. During this movement, there is a potential risk that the molars and premolars will come into contact with their respective antagonists, both on the working side and on the non-working side (Figs 6.41 & 6.42). The contact between these teeth, during crushing and grinding of the bolus of food, will determine the intensity of lateral forces on them. Such forces are potentially traumatic to the periodontal tissues of the posterior teeth.

Therefore, as for anterior guidance, during clinical evaluation of lateroprotrusive movements, the patient is asked to move the mandible from the intercuspation position until the canines on the working side make contact in the edge-to-edge position (which is in the direction opposite to the functional movement that occurs during the masticatory cycle). Again, as for anterior guidance, any interference in either direction will be manifested in the opposite direction, and if the movement takes place without any interference in one direction, the same will happen in the opposite direction (Fig. 6.43).

During lateroprotrusion, the entire mandibular body moves toward the working side. Accordingly, the inferior lateral pterygoid muscle of the non-working side contracts, bringing the respective condyle

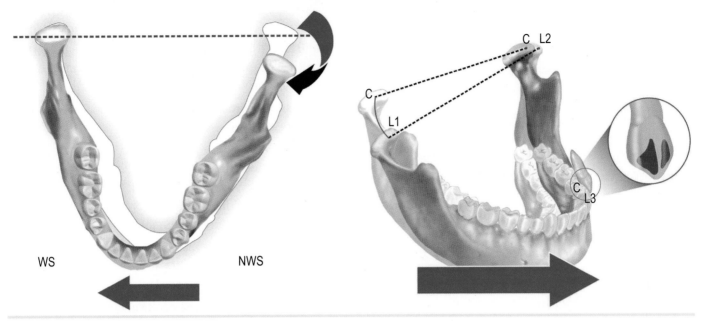

Figs 6.41 & 6.42 The side to which the mandible moves is called the working side (WS), whereas the opposite side is called the non-working side (NWS). The lateral movement of the working condyle is termed Bennett movement.

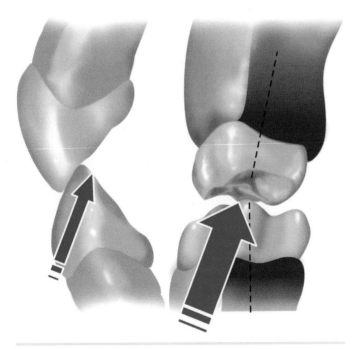

Fig. 6.43 Whatever the direction of the lateral movement, interference should not occur between the posterior teeth.

downward, forward, and medially, guided by the inclination of articular eminence and the medial wall of the mandibular fossa. The downward and forward movement of the non-working condyle leads to a larger disclusion of the posterior teeth on that side (Fig. 6.42). At the same time as the non-working condyle undergoes this extended translation movement, the mandible rotates around the working side condyle, and undergoes a discrete movement in the lateral direction, called the Bennett movement[9] (Fig. 6.41). As the working condyle does not translate, disclusion of the posterior teeth on this side is achieved by the canine guidance. Thus it becomes difficult to make a non-functional assessment of the occlusion because of the complex dynamics involved, in which the posterior teeth contact or occlude during centric closure and disclude during the eccentric movements of the mandible. During clinical evaluation of lateroprotrusion, it should be noted whether the posterior teeth disclude immediately on mandibular movement and return to the position of maximum intercuspation without any contact during the movement.

During function, the posterior teeth:

● grind the bolus of food

● act as vertical stops for mandibular elevation, as well as establishing and/or maintaining the vertical dimension of the occlusion

● stabilize the mandible via their cusp and fossa relationship in centric occlusion

● support the TMJs and attached structures against the forces generated by the powerful elevator muscles.

The anterior teeth:

● incise food

● act as vertical stops when the mandible is elevated in eccentric positions

● provide support for the mandible during eccentric movements – protrusive and lateroprotrusive – when they are involved in the disclusion of the posterior teeth

● modulate sound during speech

● contribute to facial esthetics.

Optimum functional occlusion

The morphology of the posterior and anterior teeth is easily understood. However, in a highly complex and interdependent system such as the stomatognathic system, there is a need for perfect balance between the antagonist dental arches.

In 1963, Stuart and Stallard[10] formulated the mutual protection concept or the mutually protected occlusion. This concept was later renamed by Okeson[4] in 1998 as optimum functional occlusion. The characteristics of an optimum functional occlusion are based on the least pathogenic features for most individuals in the long term. One of the major advances in contemporary orthodontics has been the clinical application of this concept:

1. When the mouth is closed, the condyles are in the most anterosuperior position, resting against the posterior slope of the articular eminence with the disk interposed. At this position, there is bilateral and simultaneous contact between all the posterior teeth. The anterior teeth also contact, but more lightly than the posterior.

2. All dental contacts generate axial loads as a result of the occlusal forces.

3. When the mandible moves in lateral excursion, adequate tooth-guidance contacts take place on the working side, discluding the non-working side immediately. This guidance is preferably provided by the canines (canine guidance).

4. When the mandible moves toward the protrusive position, there is adequate anterior guidance for discluding all the posterior teeth immediately.

5. During mastication, the occlusal contact between the opposing posterior teeth protects the anterior teeth because most of the occlusal load is absorbed by the posterior teeth.

Determinants of occlusion

For a healthy occlusion, the position, height and inclination of the slopes of the cusps and the direction of gliding of the posterior teeth must be geometrically balanced with the trajectory of the condylar movements in relation to the inclination of the respective fossae and anterior dental guidance. This balance must be present during any type of excursive, protrusive or lateroprotrusive movement. For that to happen, during excursive movements, the mandibular posterior teeth must be able to move close to their antagonists without making any contact.

From the functional and anatomical point of view, Okeson[4] considered that two categories of factors influence mandibular movements and, consequently, the relationship between the maxillary and mandibular posterior teeth during these movements (i.e. factors that influence the movement of the posterior portion of the mandible and factors that influence the movements of the anterior portion of the mandible). The TMJs (condylar guidance) represent the posterior controlling factors, whereas the anterior teeth are considered the anterior controlling factors.

The anatomic characteristics of the mandible and TMJs (posterior controlling factors) are termed the **fixed determinants of the occlusal morphology** because they cannot be altered, except by trauma and/or surgical procedures. Anterior guidance and canine guidance (anterior controlling factors) can be modified orthodontically and through restoration and prosthetic procedures. The positioning and the shape of the anterior teeth can be altered if necessary, provided certain limits are respected, so that the guidance is in a balanced relation with the directional movements of the mandible. Thus, these determinants are termed as **variable determinants of the occlusal morphology**.

The term determinant of the occlusal morphology, like most terms in texts dealing with occlusion, takes its origin from studies conducted by the gnathological school. This school focuses on prosthetic rehabilitation, in which reconstruction and replacement of the posterior teeth are often involved. However, currently, the study of occlusion has gone beyond prosthetics and forms part of almost all dental specialties. In orthodontics the term, determinant of the occlusal morphology is not suitable, because reconstruction or major modification of occlusal surfaces is rarely done. This justifies the adoption of the terms posterior controlling factors and anterior controlling factors.[4]

Posterior controlling factors (condylar guidance)

The anatomic characteristics of the TMJ can greatly influence the pattern of movements of the condyles. Although this influence can be seen during mandibular depression and elevation, it is mainly expressed during excursive movements. In turn, and jointly with the anterior guidance, this determines the way the posterior and anterior teeth relate to their antagonists and also how the centric cusps and non-centric cusps move in relation to their antagonists.

Horizontal components of mandibular dynamics

The horizontal components do not influence the amount of disclusion of the posterior teeth; however, they influence the direction of the horizontal movement of the cusps in relation to the fossae, embrasures and the cusp angles. In normal occlusion, when teeth are in the intercuspation position, that is, the centric cusps the lower molar buccal cusps and the upper molar palatal cusps occlude in the respective fossae and embrasures of the antagonist teeth. The way these cusps move, in relation to the antagonist teeth, is determined by the position of each cusp in the dental arch and by its distance from the center of rotation of the working condyle. As lateroprotrusion takes place, the entire body of the mandible rotates around the working condyle. This means that all the structures attached to the mandible have the same pattern of movement, including the teeth, which move in concentric circular trajectories relative to the working condyle. Depending on its position in the dental arch, the cusp of a tooth displays a circumference with geometric diameter corresponding to the existing distance between the tooth and the working condyle (Fig. 6.44). As each tooth occupies a

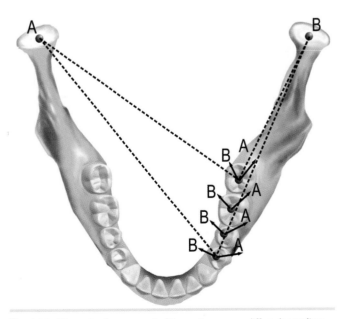

Fig. 6.44 The path of movement of the various cusps differs depending on the distance of the tooth from the condylar rotational axis. A, working condyle; B, non-working condyle.

definite position in the dental arch, the distance of each cusp from the center of condylar rotation varies and so the gliding movement of cusps also differs. Therefore, during lateroprotrusion, the circular movement of each centric cusp, both upper and lower, must correspond to the paths determined by the embrasures.

Vertical components of mandibular dynamics

Condylar guidance angle

During all mandibular excursive movements – protrusion and lateroprotrusion – as the condyle moves out from the mandibular fossa, it is directed downward and forward because of its functional contact with the articular eminence. The higher the

inclination of the eminence, the more downward will be the condylar movement. The angle at which the condyle moves outward from the mandibular fossa is called **condylar guidance angle**, and it can vary from person to person and even between the two joints in the same individual. However, in all situations, the angle determines to some extent the downward movement of the mandible as it moves forward, leading to the disclusion of the posterior teeth. The inclination and height of the articular eminence determine the magnitude of disclusion caused by the condylar guidance (Figs 6.45 & 6.46).

Lateral movement of the mandible (Bennett movement)

Lateral movement of the mandible occurs during lateroprotrusion, when the inferior lateral pterygoid

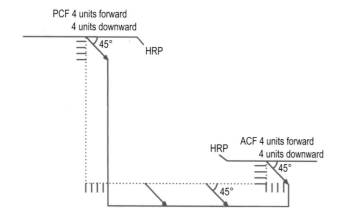
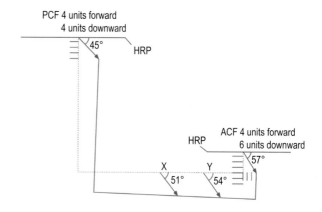

Figs 6.45 & 6.46   The anatomical characteristics of the articular fossa influence the amount of disclusion. The inclination of the articular eminence also affects the disclusion of the posterior teeth. ACF, anterior controlling factors; PCF, posterior controlling factors, HRF, horizontal reference plane.

muscle acts on the non-working condyle, which in turn moves forward, downward and medially, guided by the internal walls of the mandibular fossa, while the entire mandible rotates around an imaginary vertical axis across the working condyle.[9] The magnitude of the lateral movement of the mandible depends on two factors: the tension in the temporomandibular ligament on the working side in centric occlusion and the morphology of the medial wall (Bennett angle) of the mandibular fossa. In a situation in which the temporomandibular ligament is stretched and the medial pole of the non-working condyle touches the medial wall of the mandibular fossa, lateroprotrusion occurs in the form of a single arc around the working condyle, which in turn rotates inside the fossa without moving laterally (Fig. 6.47).

However, usually the temporomandibular ligament shows a certain amount of slackness, and the medial pole of the non-working condyle is at some distance from the medial wall of the mandibular fossa. In this case, the non-working condyle performs a pure movement toward the medial until it touches the medial wall of the fossa, and later it translates, guided by its inclination. The working condyle then begins to move laterally, while the entire mandible rotates. The lateroprotrusive movement of the mandible is determined by the amount of lateral movement of the working condyle (Fig. 6.48). During lateral movement of the non-working condyle without the concomitant forward and downward translation, the chances of interference between the posterior teeth increase because an important factor for disclusion is not in operation in the initial stage of the lateral movement.

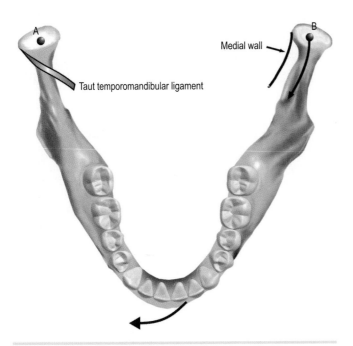

Fig. 6.47   When the anatomic conditions are favorable, such as healthy TMJ ligaments and proximity of the medial pole of the condyle to the median wall of the articular fossa, lateroprotrusion can occur without an immediate lateral shift. A, working condyle; B, non-working condyle.

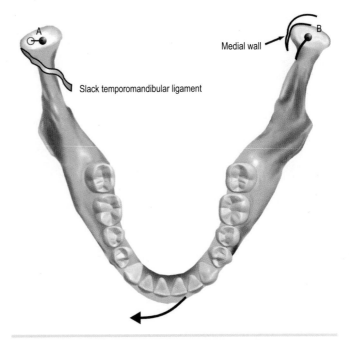

Fig. 6.48   The Bennett movement, measured in the working condyle, corresponds to the lateral movement of the mandible. A, working condyle; B, non-working condyle.

Anterior controlling factors

At the same time as the condyles descend along the walls of the articular eminences during a protrusive movement, the incisal edges of the lower incisors slide down the palatal surfaces of the upper incisors until they reach the edge-to-edge position. The characteristics of this movement depend on the anterior overbite and the overjet. The inclination of the anterior guidance is influenced by the overjet, in other words, the lesser the overjet the steeper will be the anterior guidance inclination, leading to faster disclusion of the posterior teeth. On the other hand, the greater the overjet, the lesser will be the anterior guidance inclination, and so more time will be taken for the disclusion of the posterior teeth. The overbite affects the guidance height, and thus the disclusion of the posterior teeth during protrusion. The less the

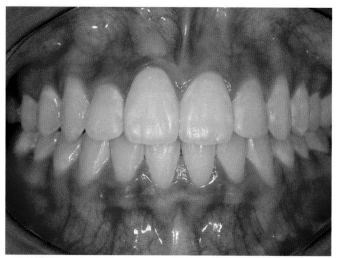

Fig. 6.49

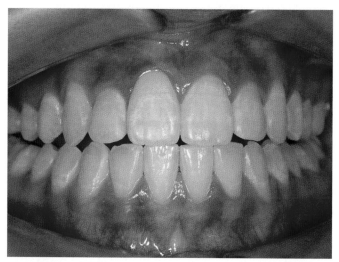

Fig. 6.50

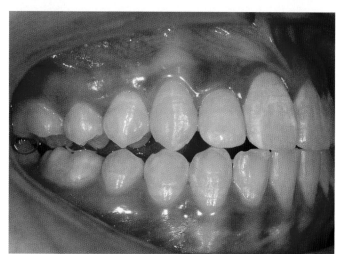

Fig. 6.51

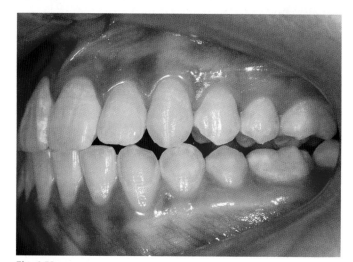

Fig. 6.52

Figs 6.49, 6.50, 6.51 & 6.52   A small overbite (Fig. 6.49) leads to a slight disclusion of the posterior teeth during protrusive movements.

overbite, the less will be the disclusion of the posterior teeth (Figs 6.49, 6.50, 6.51 & 6.52), and conversely the greater the overbite, the greater will be the disclusion of the posterior teeth (Figs 6.53, 6.54, 6.55 & 6.56).

As mandibular movements are governed by the anatomic characteristics of the TMJs and the shape and positioning of the anterior teeth, any modification in these structures can alter mandibular dynamics. In orthodontics, anterior guidance and canine guidance are important anterior controlling factors that can be altered by the clinician to achieve disclusion of the posterior teeth without any interference.

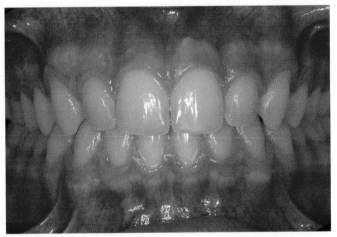

Fig. 6.53

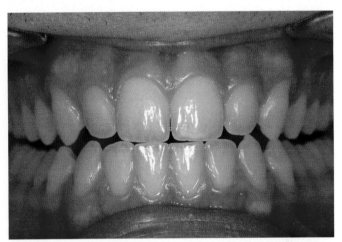

Fig. 6.54

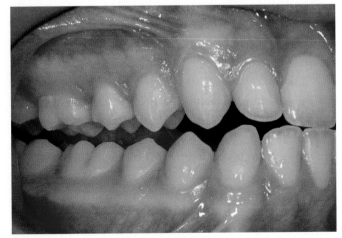

Fig. 6.55

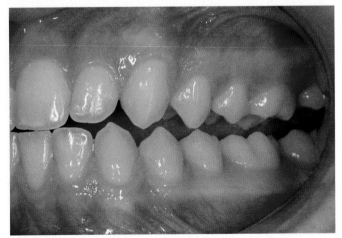

Fig. 6.56

Figs 6.53, 6.54, 6.55 & 6.56   A larger overbite (Fig. 6.53) will lead to greater disclusion of the posterior teeth during the protrusive movements.

Immediate side shift and canine guidance

The immediate side shift of the mandible increases the chances of interference during lateroprotrusive movements. However, this undesirable effect can be compensated by the positioning and function of the canines. Canine guidance can play an important part in disclusion of the posterior teeth, even in the presence of an immediate side shift. In this situation, it is necessary for the cusp tip of the lower canine on the working side to be correctly positioned in relation to the palatal surface of the upper canine of the same side in centric occlusion, that is, at a distance of 0.25 mm approximately. As a result, during any attempt at a side shift, the immediate canine guidance will be enough to provide the necessary disclusion.

The SmartClip™ Self-Ligating Appliance and anterior controlling factors

The orthodontic appliance system can change the anterior part of the occlusion, and therefore can affect the masticatory system in a positive or negative way.

One approach for achieving occlusal stability (balance) during orthodontic treatment involves establishing the functional aspects of the occlusion toward the end of the treatment. For this it is necessary to harmonize centric relation occlusion with the functional movements. To attain this, it is important to know the factors which control the anterior occlusion, as well as using a bracket prescription that will work with these factors (SmartClip™ Self-Ligating Appliance), setting up the appliance using a customized bracket positioning system, applying appliance versatility, and, if necessary, customizing the treatment by adding third order bends in the orthodontic archwires.

The SmartClip™ Self-Ligating Appliance[1] has the same tip and torque specification as the MBT™ system.[2] The prescription has been optimized to maximize the anterior controlling factors of the occlusion. Along with the use of sliding mechanics and the .022/.028 slot with .019/.025 rectangular archwires for finishing the appliance helps to establish centric relation

occlusion and functional occlusion (mutually protected occlusion) at the end of orthodontic treatment, that is, effective anterior guidance, elimination of occlusal interferences during mandibular movements and premature contacts throughout mandibular closing in centric relation.

Anterior guidance

The upper and lower incisors and canines are responsible for providing guidance during the functional protrusive and lateroprotrusive movements of the mandible. The vertical positioning of these teeth, together with their torque and angulation, must be in balance with the posterior teeth to provide good occlusal and articular dynamics.

Incisors

Overjet

As mentioned above, centric relation occlusion means that maximum intercuspation position of the posterior teeth coincides with centric relation position. Therefore, it relies on the anterior guidance.

The inclination of the incisors is influenced by the patient's facial pattern, and a balance must exist between this and the height of the cusps and the slope of the posterior teeth, so that the guidance will lead to good disclusion of the posterior teeth (Fig. 6.57). Torque control of the incisors during orthodontic treatment is the predominant means of obtaining centric relation occlusion. Deficient upper incisor torque leads to a reduction in the perimeter of the upper arch. Similarly, excessive torque in the lower incisors leads to an increase in the lower arch perimeter, thereby not allowing centric relation occlusion to be achieved.

The SmartClip™ Self-Ligating Appliance has +17° torque for the upper central incisors, +10° torque for the upper lateral incisors, and −6° for the lower incisors, that is, it has the same tip and torque specification as the MBT™ system.² This amount of torque helps with the orthodontic treatment mechanics to establish a good dental arch perimeter,

thus leading to centric relation occlusion following orthodontic treatment (Figs 6.58 & 6.59).

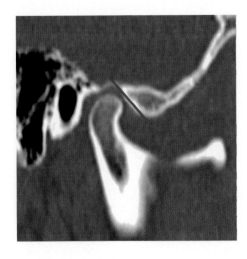

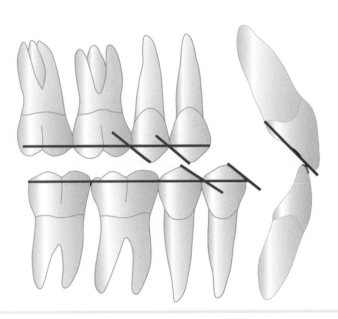

Fig. 6.57   Anterior guidance should conform to the height of the cusps and the inclination of the slopes of the posterior teeth.

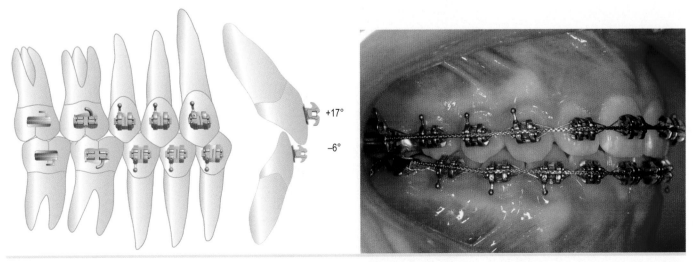

+17°

−6°

Figs 6.58 & 6.59   Torque of the upper and lower incisors and its effect on the occlusion in centric relation at the end of orthodontic treatment, using the SmartClip™ Self-Ligating Appliance.

Another factor that needs to be taken into consideration with regard to centric relation occlusion is tooth size discrepancy – Bolton discrepancy[11] – of the anterior and posterior teeth. Tooth size discrepancy can be a factor in the patient's malocclusion. Bolton discrepancy[11] (that is, excess upper or lower tooth mass), must be eliminated through enamel stripping (Figs 6.60, 6.61 & 6.62). In cases with reduced tooth mass, often the alternative is to increase tooth width by restorative means (Figs 6.63 & 6.64). But sometimes it

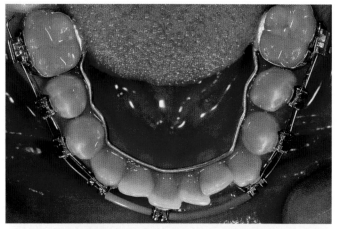

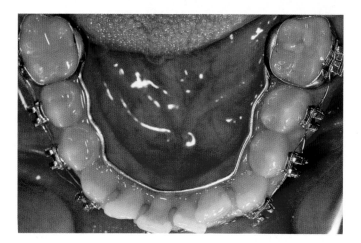

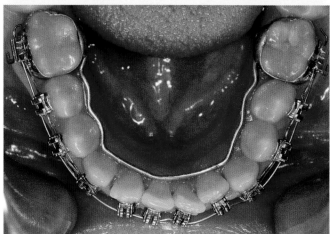

Figs 6.60, 6.61 & 6.62 In cases with excess lower tooth mass, interproximal stripping is needed to achieve centric relation occlusion. In this case first the premolars were stripped and a lingual arch placed. Then separating elastics were placed for two days and interproximal stripping of the anterior teeth was done.

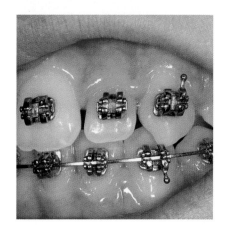

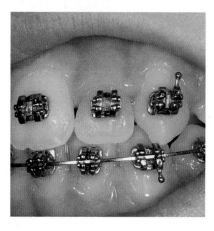

Figs 6.63 & 6.64 Centric occlusion is compromised when the upper lateral incisors are small. Composite can be used to increase the width of the upper lateral incisors to achieve adequate intercuspation of the posterior teeth.

is necessary to customize anterior torque control because of a Bolton discrepancy or other reasons. This requires good knowledge of treatment mechanics. Often what is required is upper incisor palatal root torque and lower incisor buccal root torque (Figs 6.65, 6.66 & 6.67). Such incisor torque customization allows centric relation occlusion to be achieved at the end of orthodontic treatment.

Angulation

The decreased tip in the bracket prescription for the incisor teeth, along with the customized positioning technique described in Chapter 3, allows more sound incisor guidance by increasing the contact area of the incisal edges of the upper and lower incisors. In 1998, Zanelato,[12] using semi-adjustable articulators, studied the efficiency of mandibular movements in patients in whom the incisal edges of the upper incisors were parallel to the incisal edges of the lower incisors (Fig. 6.68). The study found that esthetics can also be compromised by excessive angulation of the upper and lower incisors, because it is frequently associated with 'black spaces' in the cervical region.

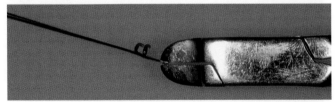

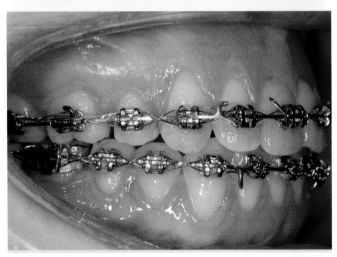

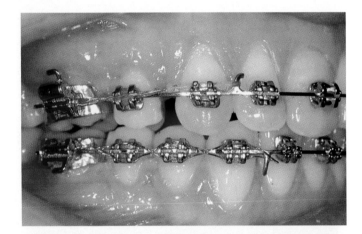

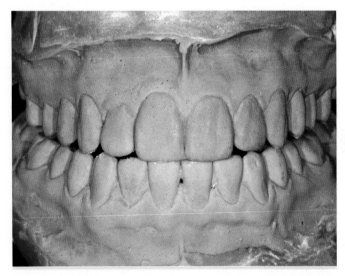

Fig. 6.68 Parallelism of the incisal edges of the upper incisors with the incisal edges of the lower incisors during the protrusive movement, at the end of orthodontic treatment.

Figs 6.65, 6.66 & 6.67 In some cases, positive torque is added in the archwire for the upper incisors and negative torque for the lower incisors to achieve centric relation occlusion. The figures show an upper premolar extraction case to be finished in Class II, with additional torque in the archwires during the space closure stage.

Overbite

As mentioned previously, anterior guidance after orthodontic treatment is related to the overjet, the overbite and the angulation of the tooth crowns resulting from the treatment. Thus use of the bracket positioning chart is important in achieving the functional objectives of the occlusion at the end of the orthodontic treatment. Looking at the bracket positioning chart, it is evident that there is a considerable difference between the height of the brackets of the posterior teeth and the brackets of the anterior teeth, and this difference determines the anterior overbite at the end of treatment.

The anterior overbite can be divided into gingival third, medial third, and incisal third (Figs 6.69 & 6.70). The

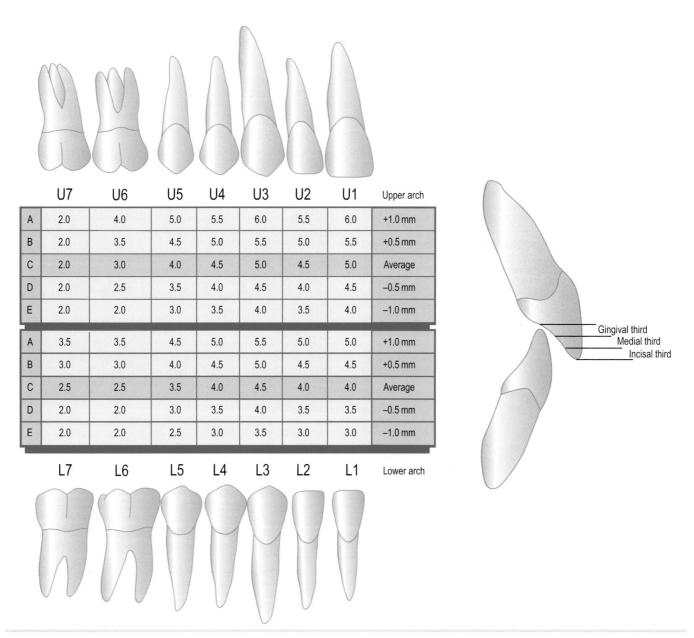

	U7	U6	U5	U4	U3	U2	U1	Upper arch
A	2.0	4.0	5.0	5.5	6.0	5.5	6.0	+1.0 mm
B	2.0	3.5	4.5	5.0	5.5	5.0	5.5	+0.5 mm
C	2.0	3.0	4.0	4.5	5.0	4.5	5.0	Average
D	2.0	2.5	3.5	4.0	4.5	4.0	4.5	−0.5 mm
E	2.0	2.0	3.0	3.5	4.0	3.5	4.0	−1.0 mm
A	3.5	3.5	4.5	5.0	5.5	5.0	5.0	+1.0 mm
B	3.0	3.0	4.0	4.5	5.0	4.5	4.5	+0.5 mm
C	2.5	2.5	3.5	4.0	4.5	4.0	4.0	Average
D	2.0	2.0	3.0	3.5	4.0	3.5	3.5	−0.5 mm
E	2.0	2.0	2.5	3.0	3.5	3.0	3.0	−1.0 mm
	L7	L6	L5	L4	L3	L2	L1	Lower arch

Gingival third
Medial third
Incisal third

Figs 6.69 & 6.70 Use of the bracket positioning chart helps to achieve the optimal overbite for the incisors. The overbite of the incisors is divided into gingival third, medial third and incisal third.

anterior guidance, as determined by contact between the upper and lower incisors in the gingival third, should provide disclusion of the posterior teeth without any interferences, and good interocclusal spacing between the posterior teeth when the incisal edges of the lower incisors contact the incisal third of the upper incisor crowns (Fig. 6.71). To have a good interocclusal space between the posterior teeth, the incisal overbite should ideally be between 2 mm and 3 mm (Fig. 6.72). If the overbite is less than 2 mm, there will be reduced disclusion of the posterior teeth, and this could lead to occlusal interferences. If the overbite is more than 3 mm, the orthodontic treatment result may be unstable if the lower incisors lie behind the palatal surfaces of the upper incisors.

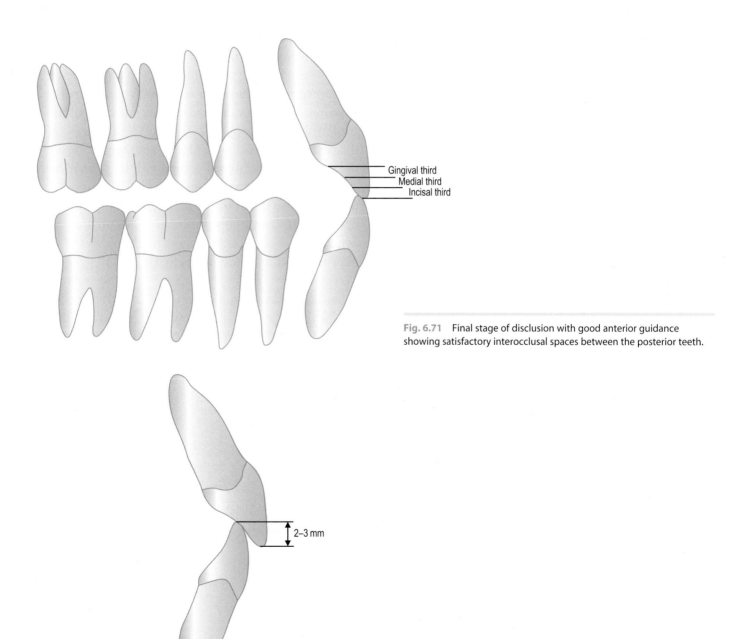

Gingival third
Medial third
Incisal third

Fig. 6.71 Final stage of disclusion with good anterior guidance showing satisfactory interocclusal spaces between the posterior teeth.

2–3 mm

Fig. 6.72 The anterior overbite required to achieve good disclusion for the posterior teeth.

Canines

Torque customization

One of the greatest challenges for orthodontics as a specialty is the relationship between esthetics and function. Besides planning for good esthetics for the patient, the clinician must also provide a stable and functional occlusion.

According to the concept of mutually protected occlusion, the canines play an important part in the lateroprotrusive movements of the mandible. These teeth are responsible for protecting the posterior teeth during these movements, and they do this by taking on the brunt of the horizontal forces that would otherwise cause damage to the supporting tissues of the posterior teeth in the long term. Therefore, good vertical and horizontal positioning of the canine crowns is a fundamental requirement at the end of orthodontic treatment, so that these teeth can perform their protective function efficiently.

The −7° torque for the upper canines and −6° torque for the lower canines in the SmartClip™ Self-Ligating Appliance is the same specification as in the MBT™ system[2] and is adequate for the majority of the cases. However, these values can be influenced by some variables such as dental arch shape, morphology of the buccal surface of the canines and tooth position. It is the clinician's responsibility to identify these variables and make the necessary compensations for correct positioning of these teeth.[13]

Canines in functional occlusion

According to Okeson,[4] the first significant development in the concept of an ideal occlusion was the concept of **balanced occlusion**. This concept was based on bilateral balancing contacts in protrusive and lateroprotrusive mandibular movements, and was applied in patients with full dentures. Bilateral contact was required to ensure stability of the dentures during mandibular movements. When rehabilitation of the entire dentition became possible, the need for a balanced occlusion in a natural dentition began to be debated. It was then that the concept emerged of

unilateral contact guiding the mandible during eccentric movements. This hypothesis suggested that lateroprotrusive and protrusive contacts should occur on the anterior teeth.

When looking at the anterior teeth it is evident that the canines are better prepared to receive the horizontal forces during eccentric movements of the mandible, because they have long roots and a better crown/root ratio. They are also encased in solid and compact bone, which is better able to tolerate the occlusal forces than the cancellous bone that surrounds the posterior teeth. Therefore, when the mandible moves in right or left lateroprotrusion, the upper and lower canines are the appropriate teeth for making contact and dissipating the horizontal force as well as discluding and protecting the posterior teeth; thus canine guidance must be one of the functional priorities of orthodontic treatment. Semi-adjustable articulators can be used for functional analysis at the end of the orthodontic treatment to check whether mutually protected occlusion has been achieved or occlusal adjustments will be needed to improve the stability of the result (Fig. 6.73).

In 2002, McLaughlin, Bennett and Trevisi[2] determined the factors necessary to achieve efficient control of the inclination of the upper canines, as these teeth have a

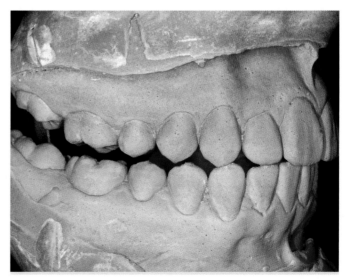

Fig. 6.73 Disclusion of the posterior teeth on the working side by the canine guidance as seen on a semi-adjustable articulator.

crucial role in a mutually protected occlusion. The objective was to establish ideal angulation and inclination for the canines, to ensure good performance of the lateral functional movements of the mandible, while at the same time ensuring maximum freedom in centric (that is, the mandible should be able to move freely from centric relation to maximal intercuspation). The inefficiency of achieving optimal inclination of teeth with preadjusted appliances is apparent when working with the canines, as they have the longest roots in human dentition. If the correct choice is made from the three torque options (see Chapter 5), the need for third order bends in the rectangular archwires will be reduced. The SmartClip™ Self-Ligating Appliance, like the MBT™ system,[2] has two types of bracket for the upper and lower canines, which allow three torque options, from negative to positive inclination for the cuspids. As a result, the position of the canines can be adjusted according to the patient's individual characteristics, as described in Chapter 5.

Overbite

The orthodontist has the ability to alter the overbite and overjet of anterior teeth – two of the anterior controlling factors. The overbite of the canines is the vertical distance between the cusp tip of the upper canine and the cusp tip of the lower canine. This distance is influenced by the height of the cusps of the posterior teeth. In other words, the taller the cusps of the posterior teeth, the greater will be the overbite requirement of the anterior teeth. Consequently, at the end of the treatment, patients with a vertical pattern will require greater anterior overbite whereas patients with a horizontal growth pattern will require less overbite for discluding the posterior teeth. In this way, occlusal interferences in the eccentric movements of the mandible will be avoided.

The bracket positioning chart recommends a similar height for bracket placement on the upper incisors and the canines but this should be customized as necessary. The author recommends increasing the bonding height of the upper canine by +0.5 mm in relation to the upper central incisor, and +1.0 mm for the lower canine in relation to the lower incisors. This change in height results in increased overbite between the canines, allowing better disclusion of the posterior teeth in lateroprotrusive movements (Figs 6.74 & 6.75).

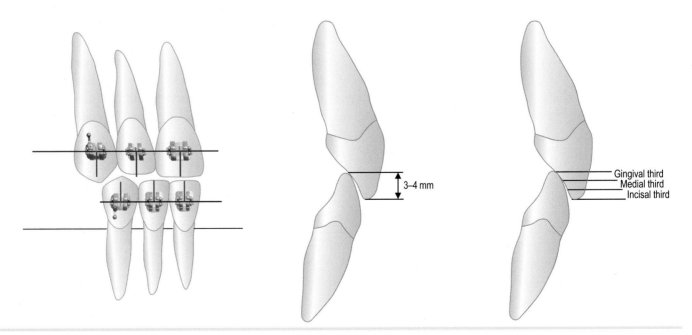

Figs 6.74 & 6.75   In some cases, the canine overbite may have to be greater than that recommended in the bracket positioning chart to improve disclusion of the posterior teeth by the canine guidance during lateroprotrusive movements.

Overjet

The overjet refers to the horizontal distance between the upper canine cusp tip and the lower canine cusp tip. When the teeth are in maximal intercuspation, the most buccal portion of the cusp tips of the lower canines must be in light contact with the mesiopalatal slopes of the upper canines, or should show freedom in centric of approximately 0.5 mm on both sides. This distance allows a certain level of flexibility during the closing movement of the mandible, and avoids unwanted contacts between the resting position and the position of maximum intercuspation. The canines act as guides for centering the mandible during closing movement (Fig. 6.76).

During orthodontic treatment, the canine overjet depends on the torque delivered by the upper and lower canine brackets and the dental arch form used.

According to the concepts of mutually protected occlusion, in the closing lateroprotrusive movement there must be contact between the upper and lower canines in the gingival third of the overbite. If the canines do not touch each other in the gingival third, it means that for part of the movement the posterior teeth on the working side or non-working side are in contact.

Occlusal plane

The occlusal plane is defined by a straight line traced from the occlusal surface of the last erupted lower tooth to the incisal edges of the lower central incisors (Fig. 6.77). Orthodontic treatment mechanics result in modification of the dentoalveolar processes, thus altering the occlusal plane in a clockwise or counterclockwise direction. The three cephalometric angles used for analyzing changes in the occlusal plane are: occlusal plane to SN, occlusal plane to maxillary plane, and occlusal plane to mandibular plane (Fig. 6.78).

Counterclockwise rotation of the occlusal plane is referred to as bite closing, whereas rotation of the occlusal plane in a clockwise direction is described as bite opening. The occlusal plane should be considered in cases where surgery is planned and there is a need to close the bite. It is also an important factor in functional balance at the end of orthodontic treatment. Therefore, the plane of the slots of the upper and the lower brackets and the incisal edges of the upper and lower incisors must be coordinated to the occlusal plane.

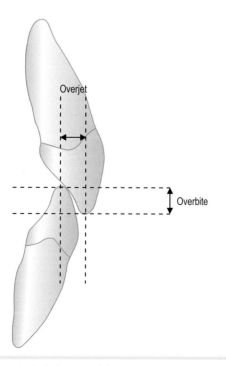

Fig. 6.76 Canine overjet is the horizontal distance between the tips of the upper and lower canine cusps.

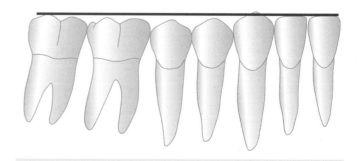

Fig. 6.77 The occlusal plane: from the occlusal surface of the last posterior tooth to the incisal edge of the lower central incisor.

Curve of Spee

The curve of Spee is defined as a curved line in the anteroposterior direction that touches the buccal cusp tips of the posterior teeth and the incisal edges of the incisor teeth. This curve was first described by von Spee[14] in 1890 as concave with regard to the lower teeth and convex with regard to the upper teeth, with the lowest point at the mesiobuccal cusp tip of the lower first molar.

In orthodontics, assessment of the curve of Spee is based on the lower arch, with the lowest point between the mesiobuccal cusp of the lower first molar and the buccal cusp of the lower second premolar serving as a reference in relation to the occlusal plane (Fig. 6.79). During orthodontic treatment planning, the curve of Spee should be taken into consideration due to the possible need for space for leveling the curve. In non-extraction cases, leveling the curve of Spee results in proclination of the lower incisors, thereby increasing the perimeter of the lower arch. The dentoalveolar changes during orthodontic treatment that lead to leveling of the curve of Spee bring it closer to the occlusal plane, thus customized bracket positioning is very important.

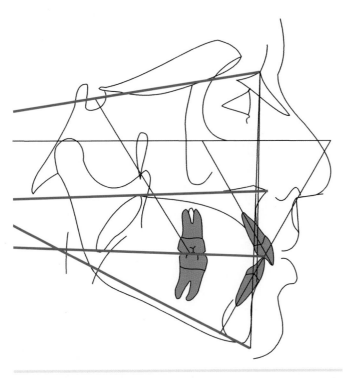

Fig. 6.78 Cephalometric analysis of the occlusal plane using the occlusal plane to SN, occlusal plane to maxillary plane, and occlusal plane to mandibular plane angles.

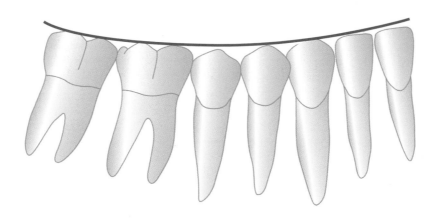

Fig. 6.79 Curve of Spee traced along the buccal cusps of the posterior teeth and the incisal edges of the lower incisors. The lowest point of the curve of Spee is located between the first molar and the second premolar.

In cases with an increased curve of Spee, the lower second molars should be included in the appliance set-up. This lengthens the posterior section of the archwire, thus helping the correction of the increased curve of Spee (Fig. 6.80). Often, it is necessary to place a reverse curve in the orthodontic archwire to level the curve of Spee, but this can result in further proclination of the lower incisors. To prevent this, buccal root torque should be added to the archwire in the lower incisor region (Figs 6.81, 6.82 & 6.83).

The curve of Spee must be in harmony with the functional movements during protrusion and lateroprotrusion. Although orthodontic treatment may be completed with the curve of Spee relatively flat, after the removal of the orthodontic appliance, there is a tendency for the curve to slightly recur due to masticatory function.

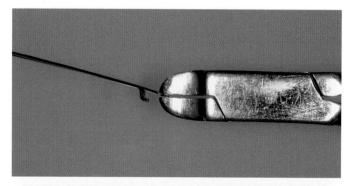

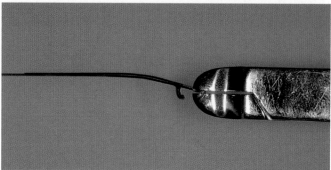

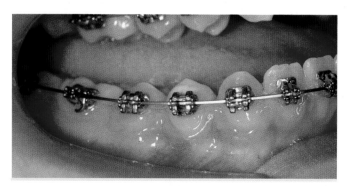

Fig. 6.80 Lower second molars should be included in the set-up when aiming to level the curve of Spee.

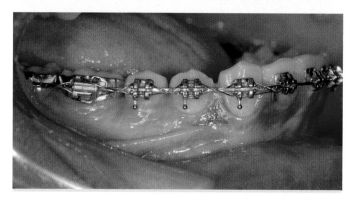

Figs 6.81, 6.82 & 6.83 For cases with increased curve of Spee, introduce root buccal torque in the rectangular archwire and afterwards place a reverse curve in the archwire in the region of the premolars to prevent proclination of the lower incisors.

Curve of Wilson

In 1911, G H Wilson[15] noted that the lower posterior teeth showed lingual inclination, which he described in terms of a line representing an occlusal curvature through the buccal and lingual cusp tips of the lower posterior teeth in a transverse direction (curve of Wilson) (Fig. 6.84). The more accentuated the curve of Wilson, the more lingually inclined are the lower molars.

The curve of Wilson is affected by the torque in the brackets and the buccal tubes for the posterior teeth. If the tubes on the lower molars feature increased negative torque, the curve of Wilson will be deeper, thus accentuating the occlusal cusps. Space closure

mechanics can also alter the inclination of the curve of Wilson, tipping the cusps of the molars more towards the lingual.

The SmartClip™ Self-Ligating Appliance features good torque control for the posterior teeth, starting from the first premolars. The brackets and tubes for the lower posterior teeth feature reduced negative torque, providing support for the treatment mechanics and controlling the lingual inclination of the molars, thus finishing the treatment with a flatter curve of Wilson (Fig. 6.85). The reduced negative torque helps to flatten the curve of Wilson, with intrusion of the buccal cusps, thus diminishing the risk of occlusal interferences on the non-working side (Fig. 6.86). In addition, the reduced buccal torque in the buccal tubes and the lower posterior brackets increase the width of the lower dental arch in malocclusions with narrow mandibular arches.

The negative inclination previously suggested for the second molar goes against all the concepts discussed above. The reduced need for negative torque for the lower second molar is related to its position at the end of the dental arch. Torque control of teeth toward the

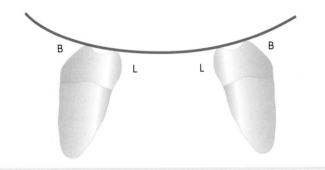

Fig. 6.84 The curve of Wilson. L, lingual; B, buccal.

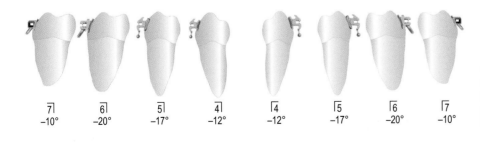

7⌋	6⌋	5⌋	4⌋	⌊4	⌊5	⌊6	⌊7
−10°	−20°	−17°	−12°	−12°	−17°	−20°	−10°

Fig. 6.85 Prescription for brackets and buccal tubes for the lower posterior teeth with progressive reduction in negative torque, starting from the first premolar.

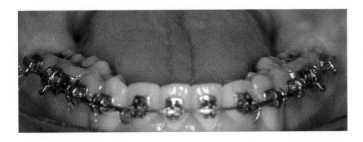

Fig. 6.86 Leveling the curve of Wilson results from a decrease in negative torque in the buccal tubes of the lower posterior teeth.

end of the arch is inefficient with preadjusted appliances, therefore −10° torque on the lower second molars is adequate.

Lastly, torque for the lower posterior teeth must be in balance with the torque for the canines for a good functional occlusion (mutually protected occlusion).

Centric cusp control

Centric cusps are the upper lingual and lower buccal cusps – the working cusps. The vertical vectors of posterior forces pass through the centric cusps, which are also called supporting cusps. During maximal intercuspation they contact the central mesiodistal grooves of the antagonist teeth, generating centric stops (Fig. 6.87).

The positioning of the centric cusps is influenced by the torque prescription of buccal tubes. The less negative torque the buccal tubes have, the more extruded will be the cusps. Conversely, the more negative torque the buccal tubes have, the less extruded will be the cusps (Figs 6.88 & 6.89). Inappropriate orthodontic mechanics can also lead to

increased buccal inclination of the crowns of the upper molars, with extrusion of centric cusps, thus generating occlusal interferences during orthodontic treatment in centric stop and in lateroprotrusive functional movements.

The SmartClip™ Self-Ligating Appliance has the same torque specification as the MBT™ system[2] and features good control[1] of the centric cusps, with −14° torque for the first molars, and −19° torque for the second molars. These negative torque values allow application of mechanics that lead to less extruded cusps, thereby avoiding occlusal interferences in centric stop and in lateroprotrusive functional movements.

In summary, the centric cusps of the upper molars and buccal cusps of the lower molars must be in functional balance with the canine guidance during lateroprotrusive functional movements. To achieve this, and for good occlusal functional balance at the end of orthodontic treatment, reduction in the negative torque for the lower molars, increase in negative torque for the upper molars, and making use of the three torque options for the upper and lower canines are important clinical considerations.

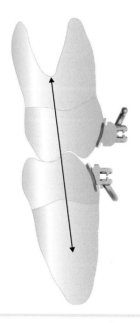

Fig. 6.87 Vertical force vectors on the posterior teeth.

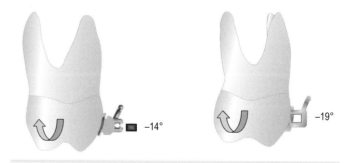

Figs 6.88 & 6.89 Controlling the positioning of centric cusps of the upper molars with −14° torque for the first molar and −19° torque for the second molar.

References

1. Trevisi H J 2005 The SmartClip™ self-ligating appliance system. Technique Guide. 3M Company

2. McLaughlin R P, Bennett J C, Trevisi H J 2001 Systemized orthodontic treatment mechanics. Mosby, Edinburgh

3. Garnick J, Ramfjord S P 1962 An electromyographic clinical investigation. Journal of Prosthetic Dentistry 12:895–911

4. Okeson J P 1998 Management of temporomandibular disorders and occlusion, 4th edn. C V Mosby, St. Louis

5. Williamson, E H 1981 Occlusion and TMJ dysfunction. Journal of Clinical Orthodontics 15:333–342

6. Posselt U 1952 Studies in the mobility of the human mandible. Acta Odontologica Scandinavica 10:19–160

7. Solnit A, Curnute D C 1988 Occlusal correction principles and practice. Quintessence Publishing, Chicago

8. D'Amico A 1958 The canine teeth – normal function relation of the natural teeth of man. Journal of the Southern California State Dental Association 26:6–23, 49–60, 127–142, 175–182, 194–208, 239–241

9. Mohl N D, Zarb G A, Carlsson G E, Rugh J D 1989 A textbook of occlusion. Quintessence Publishing, Chicago

10. Stuart C E, Stallard H 1963 Concepts of occlusion. Dental Clinics of North America 7:591–600

11. Bolton W A 1952 Disharmony in tooth size and its relation to the analysis and treatment of malocclusion. Thesis (Master of Science in Dentistry), University of Washington, Seattle, p 40

12. Zanelato A C T 1998 Functional analysis in semiadjustable articulators of the eccentric movements of the mandible in patients orthodontically treated with the straight-wire technique. Campo Grande (MS) Thesis (Specialization Course in Dentistry), Brazilian Association of Dentistry

13. Zanelato R C, Grossi A T, Mandetta S, Scanavini M A A 2004 Individualization of torque for the canine teeth in the preadjusted appliance. Revista Clin Dental Press, Maringá 3:39–4

14. von Spee F G 1890 The condylar path of the mandible in the glenoid fossa. Kiel, Germany

15. Wilson G H 1911 Manual of dental prosthetics. Lea and Febiger, Philadelphia

CHAPTER 6 CLINICAL CASE

Name: SSM
Sex: Female
Age: 12.5 years
Facial pattern: Mesofacial
Skeletal pattern: Class II

Diagnosis

Class II division 1 malocclusion with proclined upper incisors, deep overbite and increased curve of Spee.

Treatment plan

Treatment was carried out in two stages:

Stage 1: correction of the Class II molar relationship
Stage 2: detailing the occlusion with fixed appliances.

Appliance

- Headgear
- SmartClip™ Self-Ligating Appliance
- Upper modified Hawley wraparound retainer
- Lower 3–3 fixed retainer

Case report

This patient presented in the mixed dentition stage with a Class II division 1 malocclusion. Interceptive orthopedic treatment (stage 1) was carried out using headgear with the aim of correcting the anteroposterior relationship and was continued until the eruption of the permanent dentition. The corrective orthodontic treatment (stage 2) was accomplished with the SmartClip™ Self-Ligating Appliance, set up in both arches using the direct

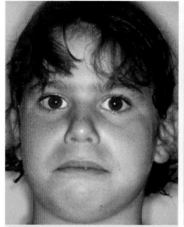 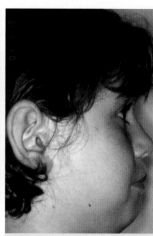

Fig. 6.90   **Fig. 6.91**

Figs 6.90 & 6.91
Pretreatment photographs showing facial symmetry, bimaxillary protrusion and inadequate lip seal.

bonding technique. The patient continued wearing the headgear appliance to maintain the Class I molar relationship until the stage when .019/.025

rectangular stainless steel archwires were engaged. During leveling, minitubes were bonded on the lower second molars to level the curve of Spee and the overbite. When using the .019/.025 rectangular stainless steel archwire, buccal root torque was added in the lower incisor segment to control the inclination of these teeth while using Class II elastics. In the final stage of treatment, .019/.025 rectangular braided archwires were placed for detailing the occlusion.

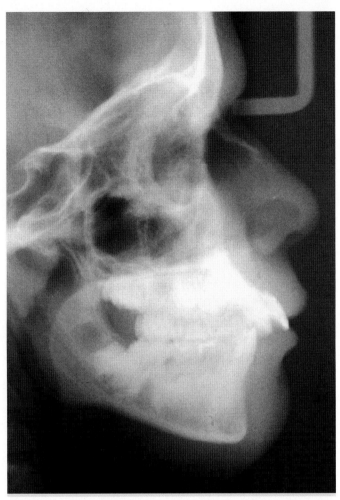

Fig. 6.92

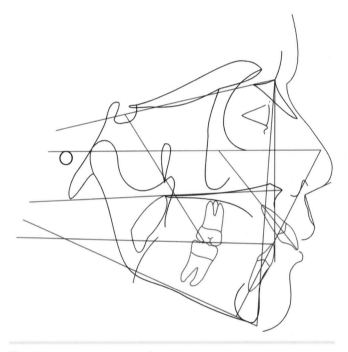

Fig. 6.93

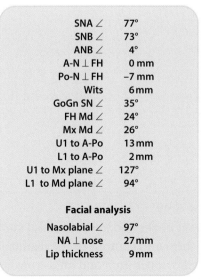

SNA ∠	77°
SNB ∠	73°
ANB ∠	4°
A-N ⊥ FH	0 mm
Po-N ⊥ FH	−7 mm
Wits	6 mm
GoGn SN ∠	35°
FH Md ∠	24°
Mx Md ∠	26°
U1 to A-Po	13 mm
L1 to A-Po	2 mm
U1 to Mx plane ∠	127°
L1 to Md plane ∠	94°

Facial analysis

Nasolabial ∠	97°
NA ⊥ nose	27 mm
Lip thickness	9 mm

Figs 6.92, 6.93 & 6.94
Cephalometric X-ray, tracing and measurements showing increased labial inclination of the upper incisors.

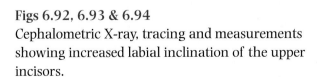

Fig. 6.94

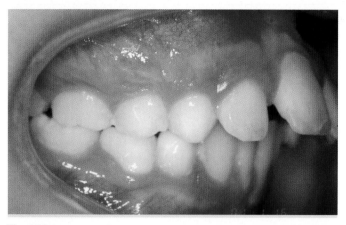

Figs 6.95, 6.96 & 6.97
Pretreatment intraoral photographs showing spacing in the upper arch, increased overjet and overbite and Class II molar relationship on both sides.

Fig. 6.95

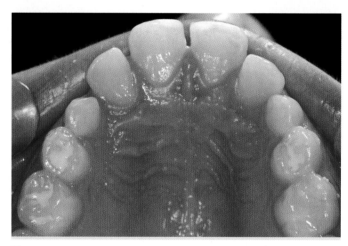

Fig. 6.98

Figs 6.98 & 6.99
Pretreatment upper and lower occlusal views showing good arch form and contour of the dental arches, spacing in the upper arch and mild crowding in the lower arch.

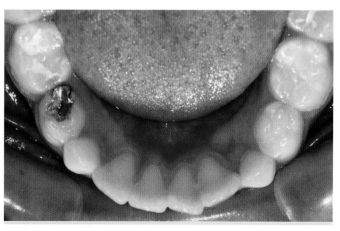

Fig. 6.99

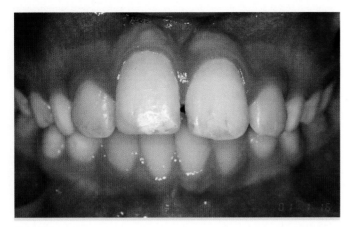

Fig. 6.96

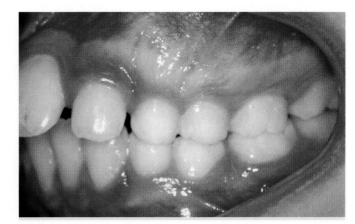

Fig. 6.97

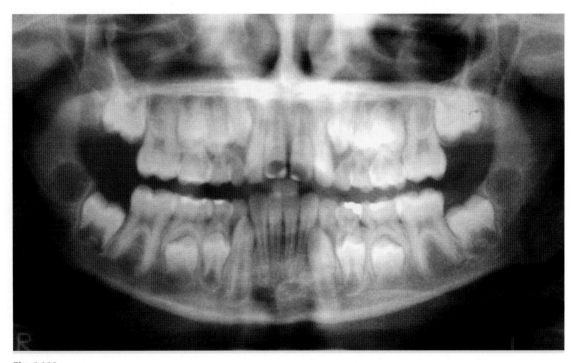

Fig. 6.100

Fig. 6.100
Panoramic X-ray showing normal eruption pattern and accentuated curve of Spee.

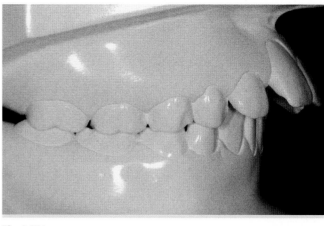

Figs 6.101, 6.102 & 6.103
Study models showing the Class II molar relationship and marked proclination of the upper incisors.

Fig. 6.101

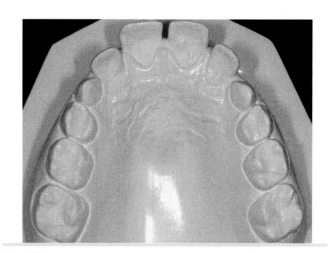

Figs 6.104, 6.105 & 6.106
Occlusal views of the upper and lower study models showing spaces between the upper incisors and mild crowding of the lower anterior incisors, but with enough space for the eruption of the canines and premolars. Lateral view of the lower study model shows the accentuated curve of Spee.

Fig. 6.104

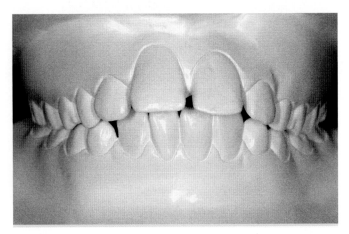

Fig. 6.102

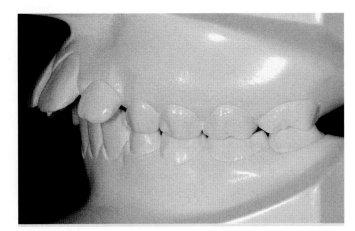

Fig. 6.103

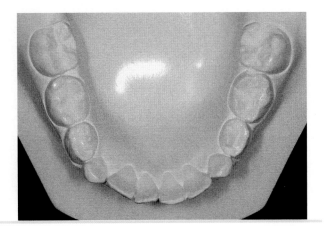

Fig. 6.105

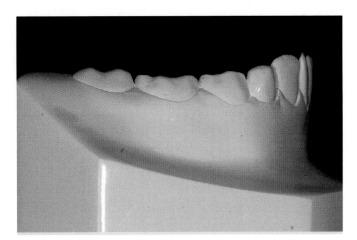

Fig. 6.106

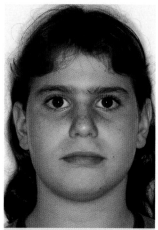
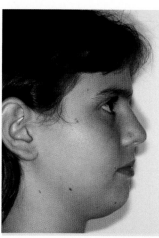

Figs 6.107 & 6.108
Interim photographs at the end of stage 1 treatment showing good facial balance. The profile view shows good lip competence.

Fig. 6.107   Fig. 6.108

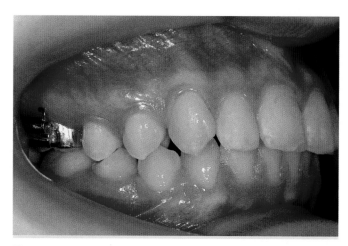

Figs 6.109, 6.110 & 6.111
Interim intraoral views at the end of stage 1 treatment showing good anteroposterior molar relationship, and an average overbite and curve of Spee.

Fig. 6.109

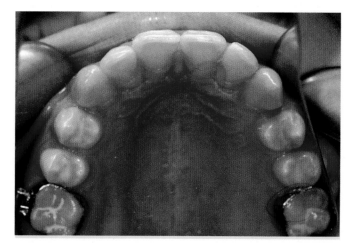

Figs 6.112 & 6.113
Interim upper and lower occlusal views at the end of stage 1 treatment. There is generalized spacing in the upper dental arch and the lower premolars are rotated.

Fig. 6.112

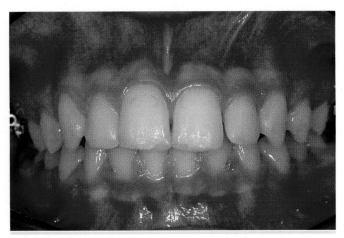

Fig. 6.110

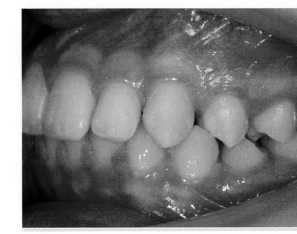

Fig. 6.111

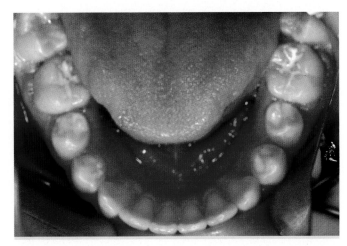

Fig. 6.113

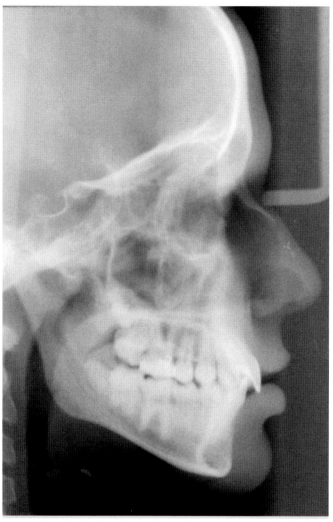

Fig. 6.114

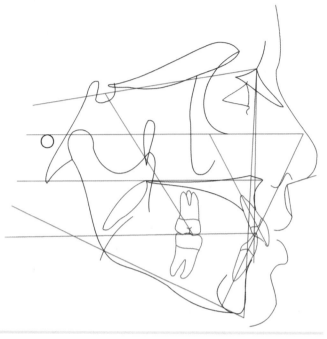

Fig. 6.115

Figs 6.114, 6.115, 6.116 & 6.117
Cephalometric X-ray, tracing and measurements showing well positioned upper and lower incisors. Superimposition of the initial and the interim tracing shows substantial mandibular growth during the first stage of treatment.

Figs 6.118, 6.119 & 6.120
SmartClip™ Self-Ligating Appliance with .014 Nitinol round archwires on the upper and lower arches. The lingual clips on the premolars are for attaching AlastiK™ modules for the initial derotation of the lower second premolars.

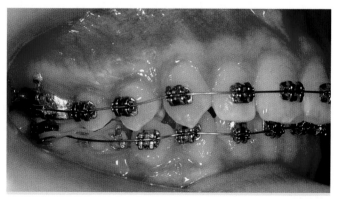

Fig. 6.118

SNA ∠	80°
SNB ∠	78°
ANB ∠	2°
A-N ⊥ FH	0 mm
Po-N ⊥ FH	−5 mm
Wits	4 mm
GoGn SN ∠	32 °
FH Md ∠	25 °
Mx Md ∠	25 °
U1 to A-Po	8 mm
L1 to A-Po	2 mm
U1 to Mx plane ∠	119°
L1 to Md plane ∠	91°

Facial analysis

Nasolabial ∠	97°
NA ⊥ nose	29 mm
Lip thickness	12 mm

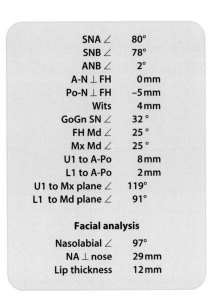

Fig. 6.116

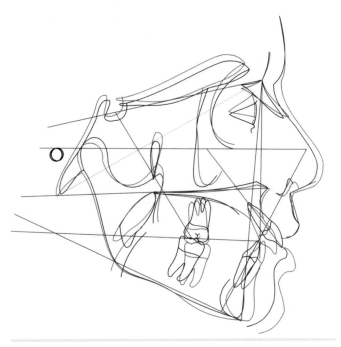

Fig. 6.117

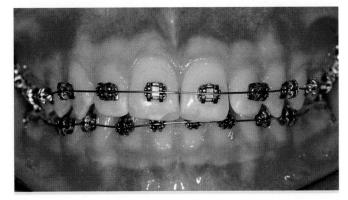

Fig. 6.119

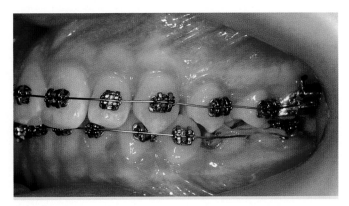

Fig. 6.120

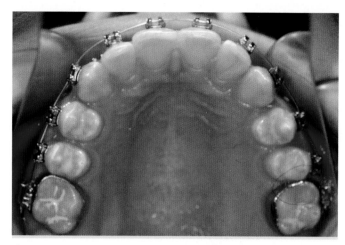

Figs 6.121 & 6.122
Upper and lower occlusal views of the .014 round Nitinol archwires at the beginning of the aligning stage. AlastiK™ modules between the lower second premolars and the first molars on both sides for derotation.

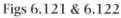

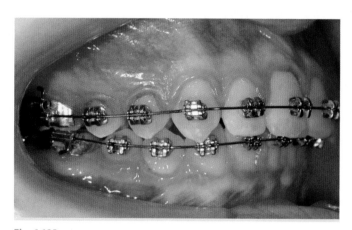

Figs 6.123, 6.124 & 6.125
Upper and lower .018 round stainless steel archwires in the leveling stage. Minitubes were directly bonded on the lower second molars to support the leveling of the curve of Spee.

Fig. 6.123

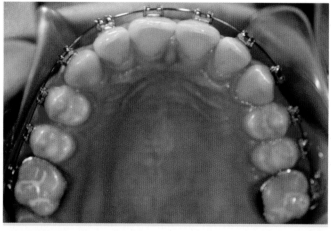

Figs 6.126 & 6.127
Upper and lower occlusal views during leveling showing the .018 round stainless steel archwires, minitubes on the lower second molars and distal bends.

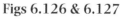

Fig. 6.126

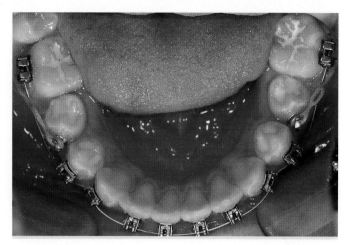

Fig. 6.122

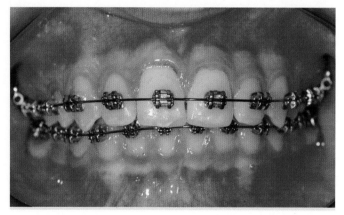

Fig. 6.124

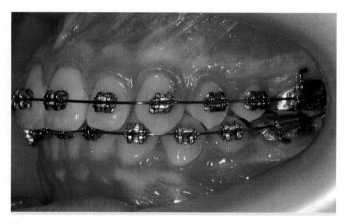

Fig. 6.125

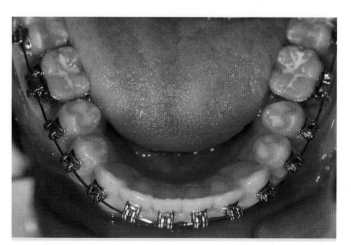

Fig. 6.127

Figs 6.128, 6.129 & 6.130
Upper and lower .019/.025 rectangular stainless steel archwires with prewelded hooks mesial to the canines, passive lacebacks, and tubes bonded on the upper second molars.

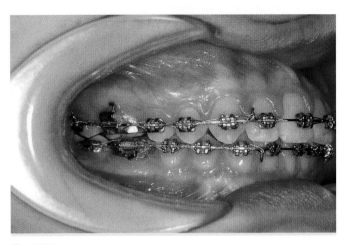

Fig. 6.128

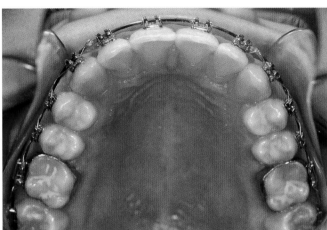

Fig. 6.131

Figs 6.131 & 6.132
Occlusal views of the upper and lower arches showing .019/.025 rectangular stainless steel archwires in place.

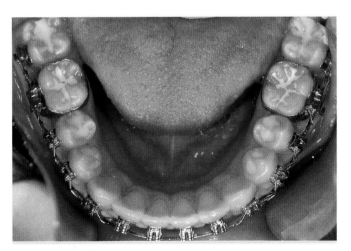

Fig. 6.132

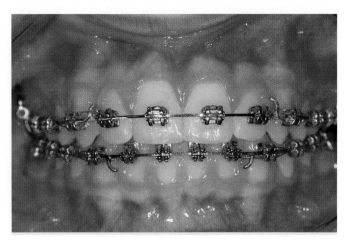

Fig. 6.129

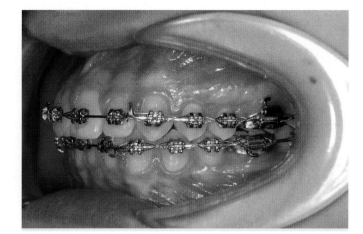

Fig. 6.130

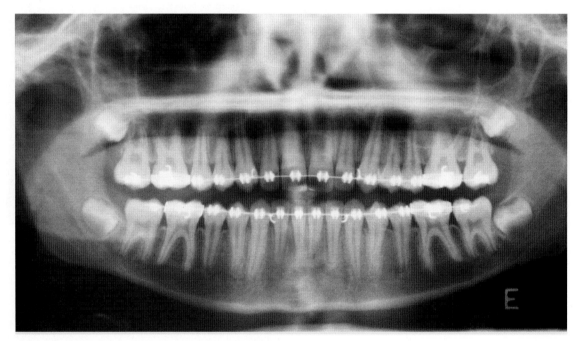

Fig. 6.133

Fig. 6.133
Interim panoramic X-ray showing root parallelism.

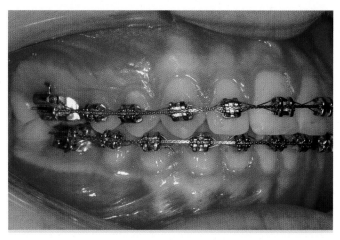

Fig. 6.134

Figs 6.134, 6.135 & 6.136
Upper and lower .019/.025 rectangular braided archwires for finishing and detailing the occlusion. The second molar tubes have been removed.

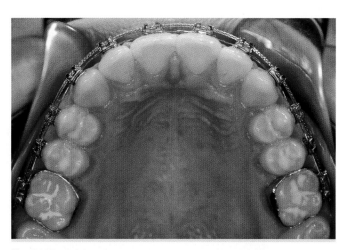

Fig. 6.137

Figs 6.137, 6.138 & 6.139
Upper and lower occlusal views showing the dental arch form and the alignment of the teeth. Frontal view showing anterior guidance achieved at the completion of treatment.

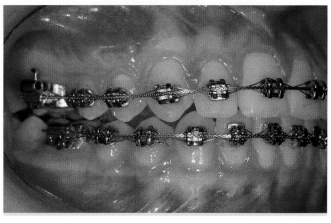

Fig. 6.140

Figs 6.140, 6.141 & 6.142
Posterior disclusion achieved with the incisor guidance: there is adequate interocclusal space in the molar and premolar area.

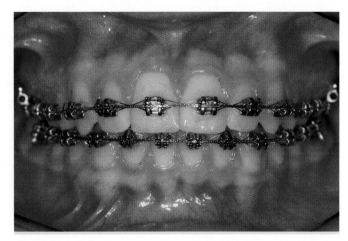

Fig. 6.135

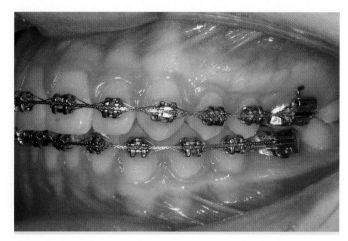

Fig. 6.136

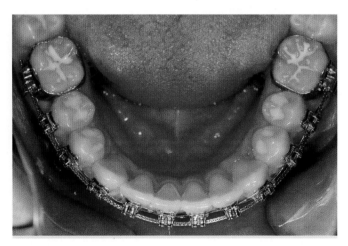

Fig. 6.138

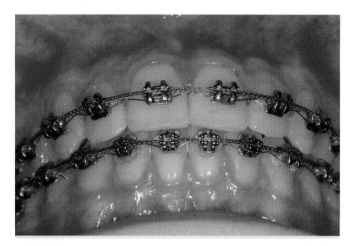

Fig. 6.139

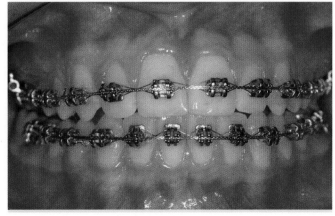

Fig. 6.141

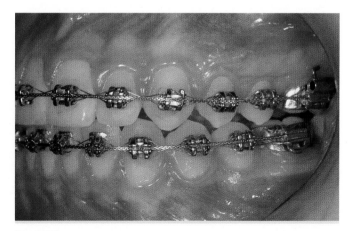

Fig. 6.142

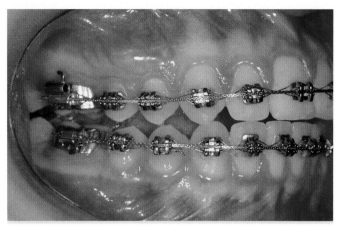

Figs 6.143, 6.144 & 6.145
Lateroprotrusive disclusion on the right side achieved with the canine guidance: there is adequate interocclusal space on both the working and non-working sides.

Fig. 6.143

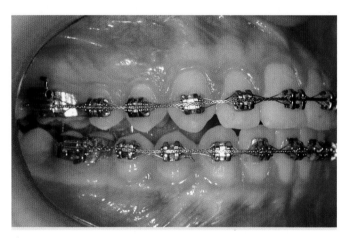

Figs 6.146, 6.147 & 6.148
Lateroprotrusive disclusion at the left side achieved with the canine guidance: there is adequate interocclusal space on both the working and non-working sides.

Fig. 6.146

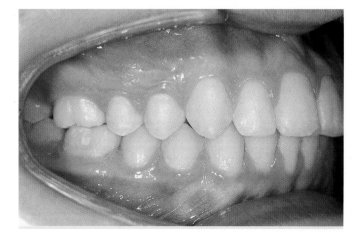

Figs 6.149, 6.150 & 6.151
Post-treatment photographs showing good intercuspation of the teeth, and good overjet and overbite.

Fig. 6.149

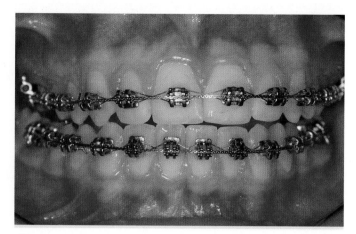

Fig. 6.144

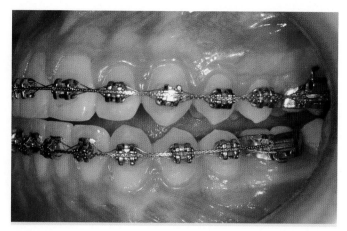

Fig. 6.145

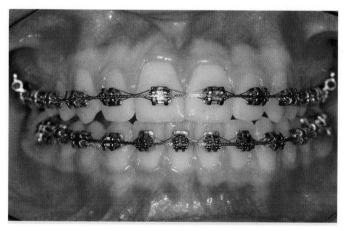

Fig. 6.147

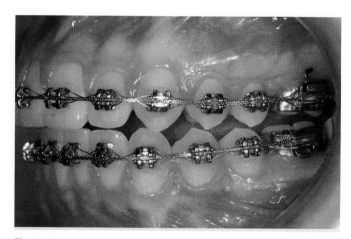

Fig. 6.148

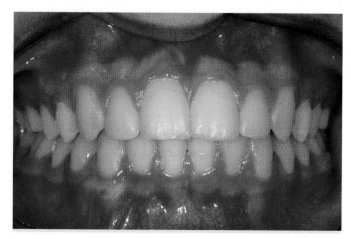

Fig. 6.150

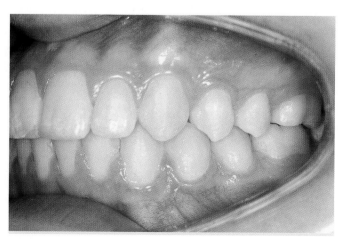

Fig. 6.151

Figs 6.152, 6.153 & 6.154
Post-treatment upper and lower occlusal views
showing the arch forms and alignment of the teeth.
The frontal view shows the anterior guidance achieved
at the end of the orthodontic treatment.

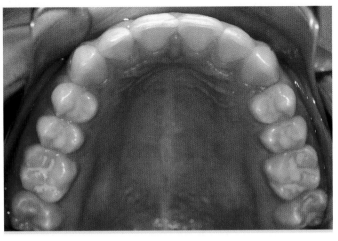

Fig. 6.152

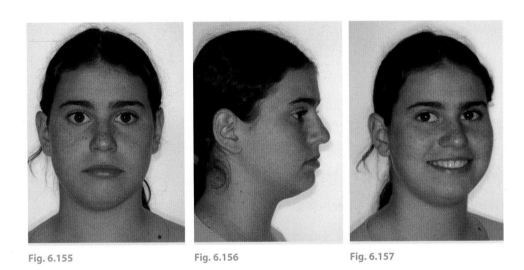

Fig. 6.155   Fig. 6.156   Fig. 6.157

Figs 6.155, 6.156 & 6.157
Post-treatment photographs showing good facial symmetry, lip seal and facial
balance. The three-quarter view shows a good smile line.

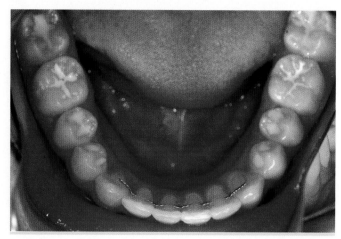

Fig. 6.153

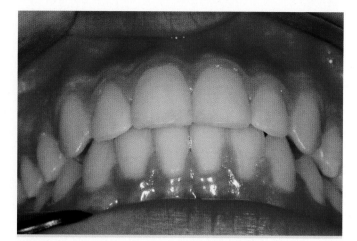

Fig. 6.154

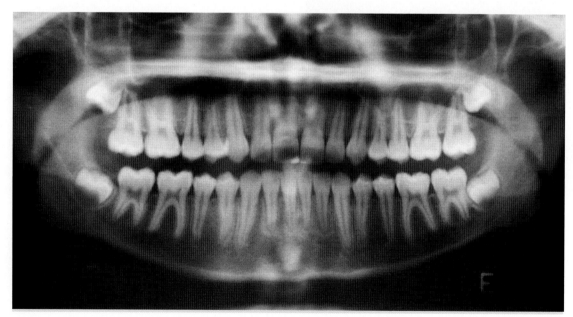

Fig. 6.158

Fig. 6.158

Post-treatment panoramic X-ray showing root parallelism.

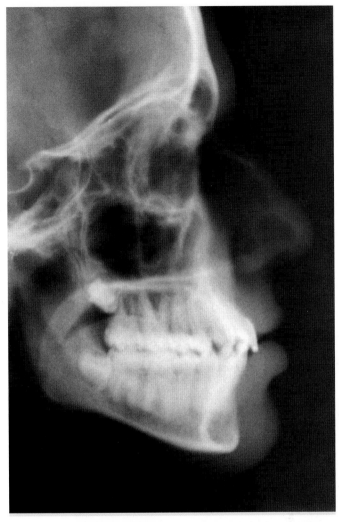

Fig. 6.159

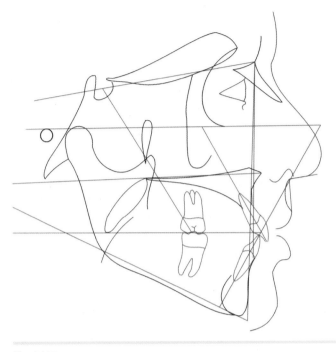

Fig. 6.160

Figs 6.159, 6.160, 6.161 & 6.162
Cephalometric X-ray, tracing at the end of treatment and measurements showing good torque control of the lower incisors. Superimposition of the initial and final cephalometric tracing shows good facial growth.

Figs 6.163 & 6.164
Computed tomography scans showing good condyle position in the articular fossa.

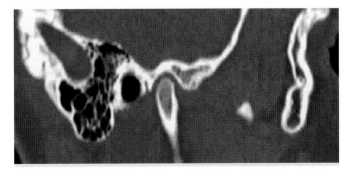

Fig. 6.163

SNA ∠	80°
SNB ∠	79°
ANB ∠	1°
A-N ⊥ FH	−1 mm
Po-N ⊥ FH	−4 mm
Wits	2 mm
GoGn SN ∠	33°
FH Md ∠	26°
Mx Md ∠	27°
U1 to A-Po	8 mm
L1 to A-Po	3 mm
U1 to Mx plane ∠	118°
L1 to Md plane ∠	94°

Facial analysis

Nasolabial ∠	94°
NA ⊥ nose	32 mm
Lip thickness	10 mm

Fig. 6.161

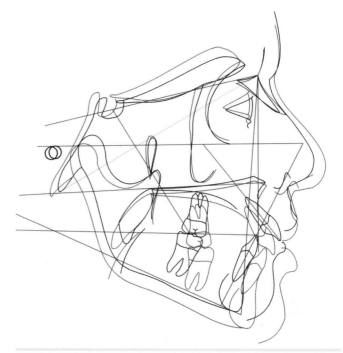

Fig. 6.162

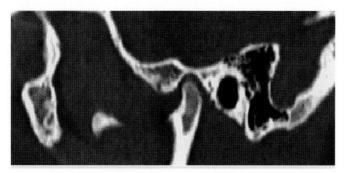

Fig. 6.164

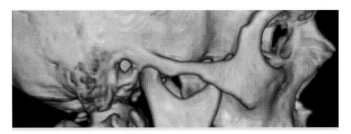

Fig. 6.165

Figs 6.165 & 6.166
Computed tomography (volume rendering technique [VRT]) showing good condyle position in the articular fossa.

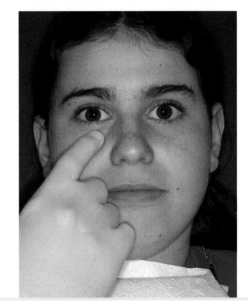

Fig. 6.167

Figs 6.167, 6.168 & 6.169
Checking the infraorbital point to obtain the Frankfort horizontal plane. Frontal and lateral views of the facial bow positioned according to the Frankfort plane.

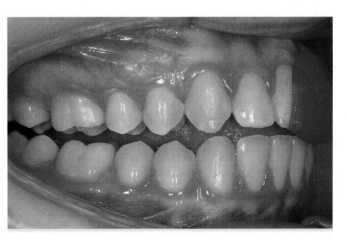

Fig. 6.170

Figs 6.170, 6.171 & 6.172
An anterior deprogramming device in position, allowing muscle relaxation and condylar positioning with precision in centric relation position.

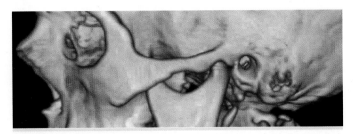

Fig. 6.166

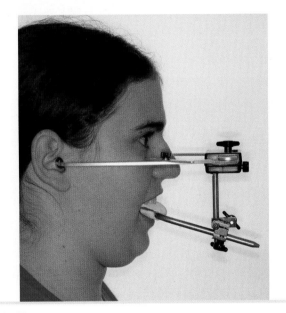

Fig. 6.168

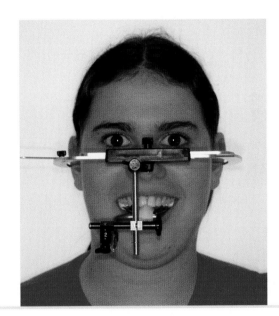

Fig. 6.169

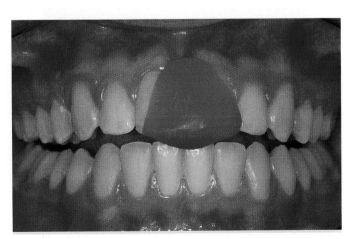

Fig. 6.171

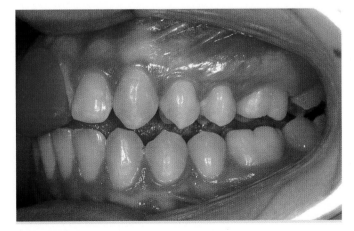

Fig. 6.172

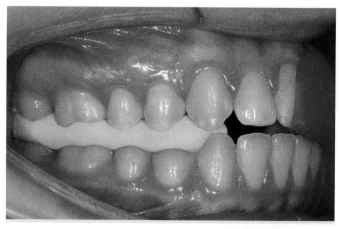

Fig. 6.173

Figs 6.173, 6.174 & 6.175
Taking interocclusal records in centric relation position.

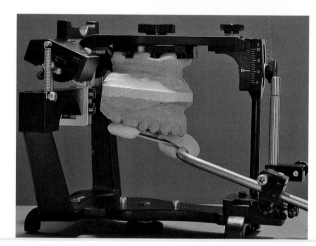

Fig. 6.176

Figs 6.176, 6.177 & 6.178
Assembling the upper model on the articulator using the facial bow.

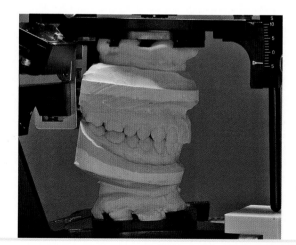

Fig. 6.179

Figs 6.179, 6.180 & 6.181
Both upper and lower study models mounted on the semi-adjustable articulator.

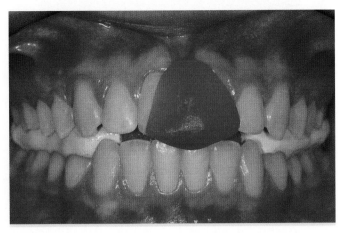

Fig. 6.174

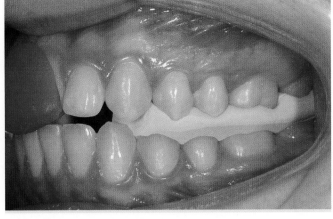

Fig. 6.175

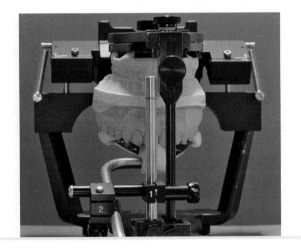

Fig. 6.177

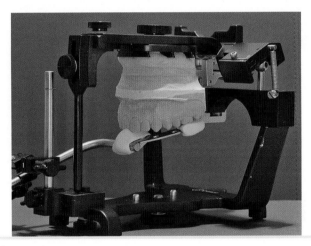

Fig. 6.178

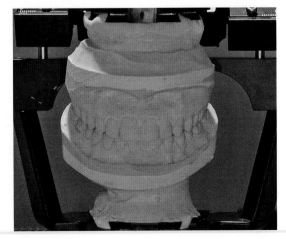

Fig. 6.180

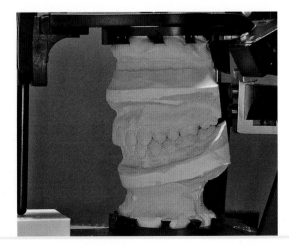

Fig. 6.181

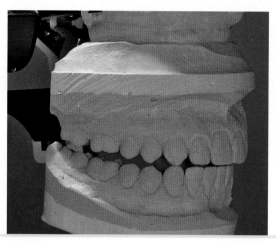

Figs 6.182, 6.183 & 6.184
Eccentric movements: lateroprotrusion toward the right side, protrusion and lateroprotrusion toward the left side.

Fig. 6.182

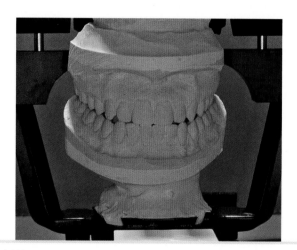

Fig. 6.183

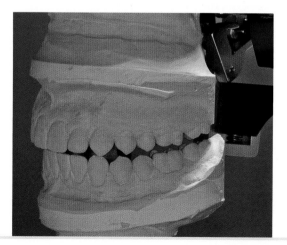

Fig. 6.184

INDEX

Fossae, mandibular 223–4
4-4 fixed retainer, lower 144
Free functional space 204
Friction 126–7, 135–6

H

Hawley retainer
  see Modified Hawley wraparound retainer
Headgear, occlusion clinical case 242–68
Holdaway 2

I

Immediate side shift, mandible 228
Incisors
  angulation 173, 231
  lower
    central and lateral bracket positioning 93–4
    interchangeable brackets 184
      axial 94
      horizontal 94
      vertical 93
    overbite 232–3
    overjet 228–31
    torque 173, 228–9
  upper
    agenesis of 186–201
    central
      angulation 79
      bracket positioning 78–82
        axial 80–2
        horizontal 80
        vertical 80
      shapes 78
    lateral
      agenesis of 177, 182–3
      bracket positioning 82–4
        axial 84
        horizontal 83
        vertical 82–3
Inclination *see* Torque
In–out values of brackets 42, 170
Interocclusal space 204

J

Jarabak 2

K

Kingsley, Norman William 2

L

Lacebacks 133, 140, 172
Lateroprotrusion 219–22
Leaf gauges 207
Leveling 131, 134–5
Lingual arch, lower 102–23, 149–67
Linguoversion, malposition 170, 171
Long gauging bands 207

M

Malocclusions
  Class I 149–67
    angulation 177–9
    Bioprogressive™ technique 10
    clinical case 102–23
  Class II 149–67, 177–82
    angulation 180–1
    clinical case 16–33, 52–69, 186–201
    division 1 242–68
      Bioprogressive™ technique 10
    division 2, Bioprogressive™ technique 10
    inclination for 182
    rotation for 182
Malposition classification 170
Mandible
  horizontal components of dynamics of the 223–4
  immediate side shift 228
  lateral movement of the 221, 224–5
  vertical components of dynamics of the 224–5
Mandibular brackets 40
  in–out values of 42
  torque 40–1
Mandibular closure reflex, deprogramming 207–8
Mandibular depression 212–13
Mandibular elevation 210, 214–15
Mandibular protrusion 216–19
Masticatory cycle 211, 220, 222
Mathieu needle holder 138
Maxillary brackets 38–9
  in–out values of 42
  torque 40–1
Maxillary expansion 177
Maxillomandibular relationships 204–22
  dynamic 211–22
  static 204–11
Maximal intercuspation position 209–11
Maximum anchorage 127, 130–1
MBT™ Versatile+ Appliance System 12–14
McLaughlin, Bennett and Trevisi 12–14
Merrifield, Levern 6
Mesiodistal angulation 38–40
Metal ligatures 138–9
Minitubes 46, 100
Moderate anchorage 127, 128–9
Modified Hawley wraparound retainer, upper 145
  clinical cases
    chapter 1 (overview of orthodontic fixed appliances) 16
    chapter 2 (development of SmartClip™ system) 52
    chapter 3 (customized bracket positioning system) 102
    chapter 4 (sliding mechanics) 149
    chapter 5 (versatility) 186
    chapter 6 (occlusion) 242
Molars, bracket positioning

  lower first 98–9
    axial 99
    horizontal 98–9
    vertical 98
  lower second 100
    axial 100
    horizontal 100
    vertical 100
  upper first 89–91
    axial 90
    horizontal 90
    vertical 90
  upper second 91–3
    axial 93
    horizontal 92
    vertical 91
Mutual protection concept 222

N

Nitinol archwires 16, 131–2, 134, 140–1
Nitinol clips 14, 36–8
Nitinol springs 139, 140–1
Non-working side 220–1, 222
Notching 135, 136, 137

O

Occipital anchorage 2
Occlusal morphology 223
Occlusal plane 236
Occlusion 204–22
  anterior controlling factors 226–36
  canines in functional 234–5
  clinical case 242–68
  determinants of 222–3
  posterior controlling factors 223–5
Omnivorous diet 220
Open bite, anterior 78
Optimum functional occlusion 222
Orthodontic retainers 144–7
  lower arch 146–7
  upper arch 145–6
  see also specific retainers
Orthopedically stable articular position 205–8
Overbite
  anterior 226, 227
  canines 235
  clinical case 242–68
  deep 78, 177
  incisors 232–3
Overjet 226
  canines 236
  incisors 228–31

P

Palatal bar, upper 102–23, 149–67
Phonetic space 204
Pin and tube appliance 3